Praise for *My Parent's Keeper*

P9-EMO-639

"Jody Gastfriend has created the ultimate GPS for family caregivers. At once humane and helpful, personal and political, she charts the long, hard, and rewarding role that all of us will take caring for our families and each other. Don't leave home without it!"—Ellen Goodman, Pulitzer Prize–winning columnist and founder of The Conversation Project

"Jody Gastfriend unflinchingly tackles a complex aspect of eldercare in each chapter of *My Parent's Keeper*. She has masterfully blended essential facts with exceptional psychological insight to create an indispensable resource for family caregivers."—Patrick O'Malley, author of *Getting Grief Right: Finding Your Story of Love in the Sorrow of Loss*

"Jody Gastfriend's clearly written *My Parent's Keeper* raises in the reader important questions about the human rights dilemma: On the one hand 'supported decision making' in which care partners—children, spouses, geriatric care managers—help people living with dementia express their own needs and decisions related to lifestyle and risk; on the other, 'substitute decision making' where care givers take over decisions in the name of safety, asserting that they know what's best for those they love and care for."—John Zeisel, author of *I'm Still Here: A New Philosophy of Alzheimer's Care*

"*My Parent's Keeper* shines a light on the conundrum of caregiving—as adult children, our best intentions are insufficient to help our parents and ourselves. We need a plan in advance of need—this book offers up-to-date guideposts for this inevitable caregiving journey."—Laurie M. Orlov, author of *When Your Parents Need Elder Care: Lessons from the Front Lines*

"Caregiving is a noble cause. The responsibilities are enormous. This book helps guide us through the pitfalls when one takes on this duty, which is both a curse and a blessing for the child caring for a parent."—Harry Haroutunian, author of *Being Sober* and *Not As Prescribed*

"Jody Gastfriend's *My Parent's Keeper* offers definitive testament to how the slow, destructive force of Alzheimer's disease disrupts generations and challenges families caring for loved ones with dementia. It is a must-read and a wake-up call to the public/private sectors who serve our aging population."—Meryl Comer, President of the Geoffrey Beene Alzheimer's Initiative and author of *Slow Dancing with a Stranger: Lost and Found in the Age of Alzheimer's*

"Jody Gastfriend's use of humor and pathos without bitterness or self-pity makes this book an easy read. The tone is conversational—never condescending, never combative—even when describing the 'maze' that health care has become and the limitations of existing policies."—Gary Kennedy, Albert Einstein College of Medicine

"Jody Gastfriend successfully weaves illustrative vignettes with practical advice to help adult children navigate the challenges of caring for aging/ill parents, focusing on potentially rewarding aspects of this often-difficult task."—Richard Marottoli, Dorothy Adler Geriatric Assessment Center, Yale New Haven Hospital, Yale University

My Parent's Keeper

YALE UNIVERSITY PRESS HEALTH & WELLNESS

A Yale University Press Health & Wellness book is an authoritative, accessible source of information on a health-related topic. It may provide guidance to help you lead a healthy life, examine your treatment options for a specific condition or disease, situate a healthcare issue in the context of your life as a whole, or address questions or concerns that linger after visits to your healthcare provider.

For a complete list of titles in this series, please consult yalebooks .com.

Joseph A. Abboud, M.D., and Soo Kim Abboud, M.D., *No More Joint Pain*

Thomas E. Brown, Ph.D., *Attention Deficit Disorder: The Unfocused Mind in Children and Adults*

Patrick Conlon, *The Essential Hospital Handbook: How to Be an Effective Partner in a Loved One's Care*

Richard C. Frank, M.D., *Fighting Cancer with Knowledge and Hope: A Guide for Patients, Families, and Health Care Providers*, 2nd ed.

Jody Gastfriend, *My Parent's Keeper: The Guilt, Grief, Guesswork, and Unexpected Gifts of Caregiving*

Michelle A. Gourdine, M.D., *Reclaiming Our Health: A Guide to African American Wellness*

Marjorie Greenfield, M.D., *The Working Woman's Pregnancy Book*

Steven L. Maskin, M.D., *Reversing Dry Eye Syndrome: Practical Ways to Improve Your Comfort, Vision, and Appearance*

Eric Pfeiffer, M.D., *Caregiving in Alzheimer's and Other Dementias*

Eric Pfeiffer, M.D., *Winning Strategies for Successful Aging*

Madhuri Reddy, M.D., M.Sc., and Rebecca Cottrill, R.N., M.Sc.C.H. *Healing Wounds, Healthy Skin: A Practical Guide for Patients with Chronic Wounds*

E. Fuller Torrey, M.D., *Surviving Prostate Cancer: What You Need to Know to Make Informed Decisions*

Barry L. Zaret, M.D., and Genell J. Subak-Sharpe, M.S., *Heart Care for Life: Developing the Program That Works Best for You*

My Parent's Keeper

The Guilt, Grief,
Guesswork, and Unexpected
Gifts of Caregiving

Jody Gastfriend

Foreword by Patrick J. Kennedy

Yale UNIVERSITY PRESS

New Haven & London

This book is an authoritative, accessible source of information on a health-related topic. It may provide suggestions to help you or your family members lead a healthy life, examine care options for a specific condition or disease, or address questions or concerns about caregiving challenges. However, neither the publisher nor the author of this book is rendering professional advice or services to any individual reader, and the ideas and recommendations contained in this book are not intended as a substitute for consulting with a healthcare provider, elder law attorney or other relevant expert.

Published on the foundation established in memory of William Chauncey Williams of the Class of 1822, Yale Medical School, and of William Cook Williams of the Class of 1850, Yale Medical School.

Copyright © 2018 by Jody Gastfriend.

All rights reserved.
This book may not be reproduced, in whole or in part, including illustrations, in any form (beyond that copying permitted by Sections 107 and 108 of the U.S. Copyright Law and except by reviewers for the public press), without written permission from the publishers.

Yale University Press books may be purchased in quantity for educational, business, or promotional use. For information, please e-mail sales.press@yale.edu (U.S. office) or sales@yaleup.co.uk (U.K. office).

Set in Janson Roman type by Integrated Publishing Solutions, Grand Rapids, Michigan.
Printed in the United States of America.

Library of Congress Control Number: 2017957269

ISBN 978-0-300-22135-0 (paperback : alk. paper)

A catalogue record for this book is available from the British Library.
This paper meets the requirements of ANSI/NISO Z39.48-1992 (Permanence of Paper).

10 9 8 7 6 5 4 3 2 1

To Mom and Dad:
With gratitude for your wisdom, guidance, and love

Contents

Contents

Contents

Foreword

Representative Patrick J. Kennedy

We are at an inflection point in history—an unprecedented stage in human development when life expectancy is almost double what it was a hundred years ago. This is a remarkable and historic achievement. More than half of babies born today in a developed country can expect to live into the triple digits. The largest growing demographic in the United States is the eighty-five and over cohort, many of whom will remain active and engaged well into their nineties. But close to half will suffer from some form of dementia. Others will struggle with chronic illnesses they may not have survived a generation ago. With this increase in longevity comes a growing need for care.

As Jody Gastfriend powerfully illustrates in *My Parent's Keeper*, families like yours are providing that care with compassion, dignity, and dedication. You are working mothers struggling to carpool kids and drive your father to the doctor. You are only children with no siblings to share or spar with. You are recently launched millennials caring for an ill or impaired parent. Family caregivers come in all shapes, sizes, and colors. What unites us is greater than what divides us. We share in a common struggle: providing the best possible care to our family members without sacrificing our own health, jobs, relationships, and well-being.

In my book *A Common Struggle*, I share my lifelong quest to end discrimination against mental illness and addiction. This mission is the result of my personal and family history confronting these challenges and absorbing their painful and powerful life lessons along the way. Although I experienced the destructive effects of silence and shame, I was ultimately healed by the redemptive power of love and faith. And I learned that care has a value. It is what saved me. It is what you, as family caregivers, provide to your loved ones every day. But you can't do it alone. The challenges you face may seem unique and private, but they are in reality shared by millions.

My Parent's Keeper takes an unflinching look at the difficulties caregivers face every day—stubborn parents, squabbling siblings, workplace discrimination, and our fragmented healthcare system. Caregivers themselves are at greater risk for depression, addiction, and stress-related disorders. If we ignore our needs as caregivers, we do so at our own peril. Yet there is a path forward and a power to our collective voice. Together, we must demand that workplaces support caregiving employees and speak up when they do not. We must insist that family caregivers are recognized as essential contributors within the health-care team and not be sidelined. We have to muster the polit-ical will to offset the staggering costs of long-term care. We must adapt technology to allow people to age more inde-pendently in their own communities. And we must demand funding for Alzheimer's disease research and eradicate this agonizing and terminal disease in our lifetime.

During my time on Capitol Hill, I authored and co-sponsored a number of bills that addressed the needs of seniors and their caregivers, including the Nurse-Family Partnership Act, the Positive Aging Act, and the Alzhei-mer's Treatment and Caregiver Support Act. We need these legislative calls to action—while recognizing that the challenges faced by caregivers cannot be met with policy initiatives alone and must be tackled within real-life families. Most of us will someday be a caregiver or need care ourselves. We cannot put our heads in the sand and hope to avoid this inevitability. We must also take the bold personal steps of acknowledging that aging and mortality should not be shunned, but rather understood and embraced.

My Parent's Keeper will help to educate and thereby empower caregivers in the trenches—sons, daughters, nieces, nephews, spouses, and partners who struggle to do the best they can with what they have. While each story is different, the burdens and benefits of caregiving have a universal theme. Assuming the care of our aging parents is an experience fraught with uncertainty, frustration, and loss. As the end of life approaches, we may feel a jumble of emotions: sadness, relief, and a resurgence of love and connection. When we bear witness to our parents' final journey from this world, we are left with their essence: memories and life lessons forever embedded in our consciousness.

I know firsthand the pain of losing a parent. Most Americans remember my father, Senator Ted Kennedy, as a dedicated, hard-working public servant. But he also was my dad. At times, it seemed that he was larger than life—that he could fight any battle, take on any foe. When my father was diagnosed with brain cancer, I knew he was facing a formidable enemy. I was with him in the House chamber after President Obama's inauguration when he suffered a debilitating seizure. I watched with reverence as he delivered an inspirational speech at the Democratic National Convention, still reeling from the effects of chemotherapy. At my father's funeral I reflected, "Most Americans will remember Dad as a good and decent hard-charging senator. But I will always remember him as a loving and devoted father." At the end of my father's life there were unforeseen gifts I could not have anticipated. Our relationship, for years often strained and distant, now became closer. My father told me of his great pride in my work on the Mental Health Parity Act. We shared moments of quiet connection. We expressed, often without words, the deep love we felt for one another. As I saw my father weaken from disease, I also saw his strength. Even as his health deteriorated, my father continued to promote causes he believed in. I share his fighting spirit. I've spent my entire career advocating for mental health and substance abuse treatment for all. I fought many hard-won battles in the Congress. At the same time, I was facing the most important challenge of my life—caring for my own mental illness and addictive disease.

My personal struggle and family relationships taught me a great deal about what it means to care and be cared for. It is not so different from your struggle. When confronted with illness and debility, whether your own or a loved one's, you must open yourself up to vulnerability and help. As caregivers we needn't soldier on in silence. Growing up, I experienced the destructive power of silence during my mother's long struggle with alcoholism. I learned to acknowledge her disease, as well as my own, and build bridges to combat isolation. I grew to understand that our collective voice is strong and powerful. What I also learned, which is echoed through the pages of *My Parent's Keeper*, is that we must reach out for help, seek support so we feel less isolated, acknowledge conflict and talk about it in ways that heal rather than hurt us. We must also be proactive and arm ourselves with information to prepare for the road ahead.

My Parent's Keeper will help—providing you with a fundamental understanding of long-term care and how to work within your own family, warts and all, to avoid common pitfalls. These compelling stories of overwhelmed caregivers, coping with their loved ones' dementia, chronic illness, and the difficult journey through end of life care, may resonate with your own experience. The lessons in *My Parent's Keeper* should be shared with family, friends, coworkers, and colleagues who are caregivers themselves or may someday travel in our footsteps. They too will join a community of dedicated people whose journeys are poignantly unique yet profoundly universal.

Preface

We don't plan for it. One day, a crisis simply brings us to our knees. Dad has a stroke and can no longer speak clearly or dress himself. Mom falls and breaks her hip. Grandma leaves the stove on again and nearly burns the house down. Whatever the event, our loved ones suffer a catastrophe and we're left to pick up the pieces.

"We" are the daughters and sons (and sometimes nieces, nephews, and grandchildren) who find ourselves caring for those who once took care of us. We are "family caregivers"—the estimated 40 million Americans who provide unpaid care to a parent or other family member. Some of us are highly educated; others barely finished high school. Some of us live near our loved ones; others live quite a distance away. Well-heeled caregivers have financial resources to pay for care assistance. Others rely on state and federal funds to supplement their hands-on efforts. But the unifying commonality among almost all of us—rich or poor, highly educated or not—is that we are simply unprepared when an age-related crisis hits us upside the head.

Most of us don't prepare for this stage of life—either a family member's aging and decline or our own. Compound that with the reality that parents may not want their children to take care of them, siblings frequently disagree on the best course of action, and the healthcare system is fragmented and complex. Meanwhile, many well-meaning adult children are sandwich-generation caregivers, juggling care of their parents with attention to jobs, kids, spouses, partners, and pets. They become crunched for time, and everything, including their own health and sense of well-being, may suffer.

But what if there was an alternative to simply waiting until you get the dreaded phone call and life spins out of control? What if you could anticipate this stage of life, prepare yourself for the challenges ahead and, at the same time, find silver linings even during the darkest of days? Those golden nuggets are fleeting and subtle and can only be cherished if you are present enough to take them in.

Part of your job as a caregiver is the painful process of accepting that you have very little control over the ultimate outcome: whether your loved one accepts help, appreciates your efforts, gets better—or not. You do, however, have control over your reactions, your approach, and your ability to remain compassionate, both toward your parents and yourself.

When my own father began showing signs of dementia, I was at a loss. My years of professional training and experience did not shield me from grief. Nor was I spared the all too common guilt that engulfs many caregivers. But I also had a compass that so many families lack. From my background as a social worker in home care agencies, hospitals, and nursing homes, I understood the healthcare system and the unrelenting progression of dementia and Alzheimer's disease. This knowledge allowed me to put a plan in place that helped my family navigate the circuitous and at times tumultuous road of caring for a loved one with dementia.

I was inspired to write this book by my own experience and the stories of families I have encountered over the years. I listened to their struggles, fears, and heartaches. I helped provide them with tools to make the best possible choices for themselves and their loved ones. And despite numerous uncertainties and burdens, these families found their experience as caregivers to be profoundly meaningful.

My Parent's Keeper explores the shifting dynamic between the burdens and benefits of caregiving. Caregiving is stressful. At times you may feel sad, angry, guilty, and resentful. But you may also experience unforeseen benefits from this transformational life passage. Caring for those who cared for you, although it brings pain, may deepen connections and offer greater insight into your own aging.

I hope this book serves as a resource for the growing number of people who make up the silent army of family caregivers in this country. Healthcare professionals, social workers, elder law attorneys, and professional caregivers will also benefit from the realistic yet optimistic perspective of *My Parent's Keeper.* With the right information and guidance, caregivers can experience gratification as they soldier on and learn to care for their parents as well as themselves.

Through real-life stories, interlaced with humor and compassion, *My Parent's Keeper* offers practical advice to establish realistic expectations of oneself and others, plan for care and its many costs, find resources to fund care, size up siblings, manage work and caregiving, and make the best decisions possible within the confabulating

healthcare system. Most of the actual names and iden-
tifying information of people who so generously shared
their experiences with me have been changed to protect
confidentiality. In many cases, I combined aspects of
different stories to create a composite that illustrates a
certain theme. The true essence of these stories, however,
is authentic and has provided the book with a fresh, nu-
anced, and ultimately hopeful insight into the nature of
caregiving. It's a clarion call to embrace the tough stuff,
the sadness, grief, sense of loss, and guilt of "not doing
enough." And by doing so, you free yourself up to seek
out support, find realistic solutions, and forge your own
path toward compassionate caregiving.

Introduction

When I was fifteen, my grandmother "Bubbie," after years of physical and mental decline, could no longer live safely by herself in her small apartment in New York City. I had very little understanding of the stress my parents experienced during their frequent four-hour drives back and forth from our house in Massachusetts to New York—trying to come up with a plan for Bubbie, who believed that a "gang" was out to get her. (Suspected gang members often included my parents.) Sometimes my siblings and I took advantage of these absences, inviting our friends over to party, only to confess our misdeeds when a stray beer can was found in my parents' bedroom. Eventually my mom and dad moved Bubbie to Northampton

Nursing Home—a relatively new facility just up the street from where we lived.

It was 1973—President Nixon had been inaugurated for his second term, Aerosmith had just released their debut album, and nobody was talking about Alzheimer's disease. My grandmother's memory impairment, frequent wandering, and occasional outbursts were classified as "senility." After Bubbie was found walking along the highway in the middle of winter wearing nothing but her nightgown, she was routinely tied to a chair with a sheet to thwart further escapades. After landmark legislation—the Federal Nursing Home Reform Act of 1987—this type of physical restraint was prohibited in nursing homes. But at the time, seeing Bubbie tethered to her chair seemed to me like just another reasonable attempt to keep my Houdini-like grandmother from escaping. The nursing home had previously tried plastering signs on all the exits that read: "Celia Swing [my Bubbie], Do Not Enter!" Given that my grandmother mainly spoke Yiddish and was unlikely to read signs anyway, this strategy, like many others, proved futile.

Fast-forward thirty-eight years. I am now fifty-three. I vividly remember my frequent visits to Bubbie in the nursing home. I would leave my Raleigh in the bicycle rack in the parking lot. Now, struck by the bizarre set of circumstances that once again brings me to this place, I pull my car into one of the vacant spaces in that very same parking lot. When I walk into the building, I immediately notice the faint institutional odor of antiseptic and bodily fluids. I take the elevator to the second floor, turn right, and go through the double doors. The unit looks strikingly similar to the way it looked years ago. I imagine my Bubbie sitting in her chair near the nursing station. I turn left down the corridor and enter a small room with a freshly made bed and a cheerfully decorated window looking out over my old neighborhood. In a wheelchair a man sits hunched over in what appears to be a light, peaceful slumber. "Dad," I say softly as I lightly touch his shoulder. "It's me—Jody—your daughter." My father's eyes open slowly, and he looks up at me with a tentative flash of recognition. A few seconds pass. Then my dad smiles sweetly and gently takes my hand.

That was a year before my father died—toward the end of our family's long caregiving odyssey. As a social worker with over twenty-five years of experience in the eldercare field and as an adult child of a father with progressive dementia, I know the burdens and uncertainties that caregivers face every day. I understand the difficulties of juggling my own family and work responsibilities with the demands of caring for a parent who cannot care for himself. I have heard the stories of hundreds of people like me, who find themselves in a role they did not anticipate or prepare for. At various times isolated, uncertain, sad, and hopeful, family caregivers move forward with compassion and strength. Family caregivers, people like you and me, are the centerpiece of our nation's system of long-term care.

Over the years, my family struggled with many difficult decisions regarding my father's care. We faced numerous obstacles within the healthcare system, and tried to balance my father's needs with my mother's ability to care for him safely at home. Eventually we made the difficult decision to place my father in a nursing home.

Making effective decisions about the care of a loved one often takes more time than anticipated. It requires an understanding of the long-term care system that many people lack. The average caregiver spends over twenty hours per week on activities such as bathing, dressing, housework, errands, managing finances—and the list goes on. Caregivers have these responsibilities for an average of four years—and significantly longer if they are caring for a loved one with dementia. This is a marathon, not a sprint. To properly run a marathon, you need preparation to go the distance and get past the heartbreak hills that are just around the bend.

Our family was fortunate in many ways. My mother, who visited my father every day in the nursing home, found ways to remain engaged with my dad through storytelling, reminiscing, humor, and imagination. My father's kindness, loving nature, and remarkable ability to live in the moment helped us accept the many losses he endured and instead focus on what remained. As my father bravely struggled to retain his personhood, he taught us that quality of life can persevere and the ability to love need not be extinguished by a devastating illness.

Being truly present with a loved one has helped many families like mine accept the inevitable losses that are an undeniable part of this life journey. Although a tactical approach to caregiving is essential in providing the knowledge and tools to make informed decisions, caregiving is so much more than checklists and roadmaps. It is an opportunity to redefine your relationships with elder parents, learn from them as they endure chronic illness and the infirmities of old age, and embrace the precious time you have together.

Caregiving is also about holding on and letting go. We must focus on the demands of the present and find ways to honor the past. We also have the task of bearing witness to memory, an intangible link that connects us to the generations that came before us. Since the death of my father, I hold on dearly to the many stories that express the spirit of the man he once was, that capture his essence. As caregivers, we carry these legacies within our hearts, in the hope that the memory of our loved ones will continue to live on, long after they are gone.

ONE

The Journey Begins

We don't receive wisdom; we must discover it
for ourselves after a journey that no one can
take for us or spare us.
—MARCEL PROUST

"Where is Dad?" I remember asking as my family and I were leaving the synagogue after High Holiday services. I searched the library and classrooms as my brother checked the men's room. We asked family friends if they had seen my father, but no one had a clue where he'd gone. It was a beautiful fall day in western Massachusetts. The leaves had barely changed their hue and there was just a hint of coolness in the air. Could my father have taken advantage of the glorious weather and gone for a stroll? But why would he wander off without telling anyone? My mother's initial response to my father's disappearance was anger. Didn't Dad know that we were planning a big holiday meal? As time slowly passed without any sign of my father, the anger dissipated and was replaced by a stomach-churning anxiety. And then he emerged from the woods that marked the perimeter of the bike path, a converted railroad track that had become a haven for joggers and cyclists. My father, in his suit and tie that a few hours earlier had looked so dapper, now appeared disheveled, agitated, and confused.

"Dad, where've you been? We've been looking all over for you," I said. In an angry tone, my father replied incomprehensibly, "I went to pick up the dry cleaning!" While my father enjoyed his weekly errands, walking off during a holiday to pick up laundry without telling anyone made absolutely no sense and was a worrisome omen. That incident marked the beginning of a long odyssey into a world many families know all too well—caring for a loved one with dementia. Looking back, we could recognize earlier signs, like missed appointments and unpaid bills. While we attributed some slip-ups to my dad's absent-minded professor persona, when it came to appointments and bills, he had always been precise. With a PhD in psychology, my father was both educated and worldly. He had an incredible fund of knowledge and a mastery of world geography. Even with dementia, my father could recall Otto von Bismarck's contribution to the German Empire in the nineteenth century. But he couldn't remember what he'd had for lunch.

For many families like mine, it may be tempting to ignore early signs of dementia. The realization that a parent, spouse, partner, or other loved one has a devastating disease that can rob them of their most fundamental capabilities can be too much to bear. We attribute memory lapses and mood changes to old age rather than illness. But old age is a stage of life, not a disease. Many people, like my mother, are active and engaged well into their eighties and beyond. People can continue to grow, learn, and love even with dementia, as my dad so movingly showed us.

So when should you be concerned about your mother's memory lapses? Or your father's driving? Perhaps your grandmother forgets the recipe of the same apple pie she has made for thirty years. Or your fastidious uncle can no longer manage his personal hygiene. Not long after the incident at the synagogue, my father got lost driving home from the post office, a trip he had taken thousands of times. We had to come to grips with a harsh reality—what would soon become our "new normal." Recognition of my father's cognitive decline was the first step in a very arduous and unpredictable journey—one that, despite its many losses and burdens, would teach us unexpected life lessons.

Warning Signs

Families often dismiss the early warning signs, as we did, until the alarm grows louder. When what was once familiar becomes jarringly unfamiliar, it can be frightening. The most mundane tasks, such as cooking, going to the bathroom, managing finances, or driving, perilously shift from routine to high risk. In some cases, a loved one no longer recognizes a spouse or child. My father, before Google maps and GPS, could arrive in a foreign country and easily find his way from airport to hotel. Now he would get lost on familiar routes and was no longer safe behind the wheel. And my mother, who never paid a bill throughout her married life, had to take over the finances.

While initially my family struggled to acknowledge my father's disease, incredibly, he did not. "I think I am becoming senile," my dad would say after an incident when he could not retrieve some detail from his day. While this saddened my father, he chose not to fight it. My father's unusual ability to accept his dementia was an unforeseen gift, one that helped our family deal with the inevitable guilt and grief to follow.

Crossing a Threshold

For many families, a diagnosis of dementia can bring on a whirlwind of emotions: anger, denial, and profound sadness, both for the caregiver and the loved one with the disease. In addition, there will be a lot of practical questions: Where can I find the right care? What do I need to know about the disease? How can I get support as a caregiver? A great resource is the Alzheimer's Association® (www.alz.org). The Alzheimer's Association works on a global level to support those affected by Alzheimer's disease and other dementias and has local chapters that identify resources within a community. The organization also offers a professionally staffed 24/7 helpline, providing information and advice in more than two hundred languages.

Receiving a diagnosis of Alzheimer's disease is devastating, but knowing the truth can also reduce confusion and provide much-needed answers. That was the case with Steven, a computer engineer for a multinational technology company and the only child of immigrant parents from South Korea. Steven was concerned about his father, who was beginning to forget names and repeat stories. When his father reported the car stolen after misplacing it in a parking garage, Steven became seriously alarmed. A host of other warning signs followed, such as unread mail, mix-ups with medication, and repeated difficulty recalling words. "I was beginning to feel that my father was no longer safe at home. My dad was a proud, stubborn man and he would become angry when I suggested any help, so I backed off." Steven's frustrations were compounded by his complicated relationship with his father, who had been a harsh disciplinarian. "My father was easily angered and his flare-ups would intimidate me. My mother's easygoing nature provided a balance. She was both buffer and caregiver." She relied greatly on Steven, her only respite, to step in when a crisis erupted. And it inevitably did. After Steven's father locked himself out of the house one day, he became disoriented, wandering for hours in the cold. Finally, a neighbor found him and called the police. Steven's mother was despondent, which only reinforced Steven's feelings of helplessness: "I felt like I was riding a train without a conductor that could be derailed at any moment."

Feeling helpless, not knowing how to aid and protect the person who raised you, no matter how imperfectly, is one of the more agonizing aspects of caring for aging parents. Your ability to alleviate their pain and suffering is limited. You have no control over how events will unfold. But you can make a difference—by getting the right information, putting a plan of care in place, and forging ahead despite setbacks and sorrows. In the early stages of this journey, when you are grappling with the realization that something has changed and you've crossed a threshold, you are in mourning. You know you can't go back to being the cared-for child and instead must assume the role of caregiver. As Steven said, "My parents were always my safety net. I don't have that anymore. Now I am the net."

Seek Medical Advice—Easier Said Than Done

One of the first recommendations I make for people in Steven's situation is to seek a medical evaluation for their parent early on, ideally with a geriatrician. This eliminates some of the guesswork that comes from trying to figure out a solution to a problem that has yet to be defined. Geriatricians, doctors who specialize in the care of older adults, are in great demand and not so easy to find. And it is getting tougher. According to the American Geriatric Society, ideally, there should be one geriatrician available for every seven hundred patients. But that is far from the case. Today there are only about seven thousand certified geriatricians in the United States—one for every twenty-six hundred older Americans.[1] By 2050, the U.S. population of people sixty-five or older will be close to double what it is today. Globally, the number is expected to nearly triple. The shortage of healthcare providers who are trained to treat the multiple chronic conditions that afflict this aging population will continue to be a vexing challenge.

Charlotte Grinberg, a fourth-year medical student with a passion for working with older adults, is a bit of an anomaly. Out of a medical school class of 270 students, Charlotte was one of only four who chose to do an optional rotation in geriatrics. Growing up, Charlotte was very close to her grandparents and witnessed the challenges they faced navigating an indifferent healthcare system. That inspired Charlotte to pursue a career caring for older people—a desire not generally shared by her contemporaries. "I just don't see appreciation for aging among my peers in medicine," says Charlotte. "The second I express my interest in geriatrics, my colleagues cringe." Currently, 97 percent of all medical students in the United States do not take a single course in geriatrics.[2] They certainly are not flocking to this underpaid and not-so-sexy subspecialty.

Many primary care physicians, particularly in communities with a high percentage of seniors, already have significant experience caring for an aging patient population. While they may not be geriatricians, they are a good place to start and can direct you to memory disorder clinics, often located within hospitals and healthcare systems, where your parent can get an accurate diagnosis and a recommended plan of care.

Of course, convincing someone to see a doctor is another issue. Steven's coercive efforts to get his father to see a doctor, not surprisingly, met some resistance. Our parents should be partners in the endeavors we undertake to get them the help they need but don't necessarily want. We can provide information, guidance, and support. But as long as our parents are medically competent to make decisions, they hold the reins. So Steven lightened his approach and replaced stern admonishments with gentle coaxing. He engaged his father in the process, including scheduling the appointment at a memory disorder clinic, giving Steven's father some semblance of control. Following a thorough assessment, Steven learned his father was suffering from Alzheimer's disease. Steven was devastated. He was also relieved. In caregiving, these feelings are not mutually exclusive—they often coexist. "As odd as it may seem, getting the diagnosis was empowering," Steven explained. "Dealing with the unknown was worse." Steven had felt powerless to take action when he was responding mostly to fear rather than facts.

By the time we took my father to the memory disorder clinic at Massachusetts General Hospital, most of our denial had ebbed away. The psychiatrist who evaluated my dad, Dr. William Falk, was a colleague of my husband's (also a psychiatrist at MGH). Dr. Falk was someone I knew and trusted. He was knowledgeable, kind, and empathic—qualities that are tough to find within the modern healthcare system. It was 1998; I had just turned forty and was feeling the weight of impending middle age. My mother, not yet seventy, was stoic and brave. We braced ourselves as the doctor delivered his findings. We knew what was coming. My father listened attentively to the explanation of the disease that was chipping away at his beautiful mind. I held his hand and cried as he nodded with pained acceptance.

Acceptance

In her landmark book *On Death and Dying*, the Swiss psychiatrist Dr. Elisabeth Kübler-Ross outlined a framework for understanding the emotional stages of grief and loss that are a natural reaction to death.[3] This model can also be applied to major life events—divorce, unemployment, addictions, and the life-altering realization that you or your loved one has a debilitating disease such as dementia. From denial to acceptance, Kübler-Ross gave us a glimpse into the messy emotional terrain we all must traverse when we face life's losses. Getting to a place where we can accept what *is* and not just lament what *isn't* means that we first must experience—and even embrace—our own sadness.

Consider *Inside Out*, Pixar's brilliant and psychologically sophisticated film about the emotional life of an eleven-year-old girl experiencing the loss of friends and family cohesion when she moves to a new city. The film deftly portrays the interdependent connection between joy and sadness. The emotions are actually characters in the movie, and they often engage in antic struggles to assert their superiority. But it is sadness that ultimately saves the day, balancing the repressive intensity of joy's feigned cheerfulness in the face of loss. Only when sadness is given voice and pain is acknowledged can the healing truly begin.

Steven learned that lesson from his caregiving experience. As a computer engineer, Steven was generally more comfortable processing data than feelings. Friends described him as a lovable Vulcan. But Steven ultimately acknowledged his sadness, which allowed him to mourn the strong, powerful father he had known and accept the more vulnerable and helpless man he was struggling to understand. The flood of emotion he experienced as his father grew increasingly frail unnerved Steven. "I did not have the language to describe what was happening. I felt exhausted, angry, and disinterested. In retrospect, I was depressed but didn't know it." After the diagnosis, Steven reached out to a social worker through an eldercare benefit offered by his employer. The social worker helped Steven find a caregiver support group. At first the stories others shared were too close to home and their sadness was overwhelming. But in time, Steven found the group to be a much-needed anchor in a sea of uncertainty and turbulence. Reflecting on the experience, Steven explains: "I tell people in stressful caregiving situations that the emotions they are experiencing—sadness, fear, anxiety, anger, frustration—are all normal reactions to a difficult situation. People need to be reassured that it's okay and that it is part of being human. At the same time, that bit of self-awareness helped me cope with what I was experiencing and steer my energy in a productive and positive direction."

Once Steven came to terms with his father's diagnosis, he stopped fighting. "Before I accepted that, I was fighting a lot. It was all a fight. Once I understood this was really happening, I accepted that I was now a caregiver. This is the new reality. I have to figure out what is going on and adjust to it. And keep adjusting. I could not be focused on healing old wounds."

Make Contingency Plans

It has been said, "People don't plan to fail. They fail to plan." Several years ago my mother posed a difficult question to my siblings and me: "What if I were to die before your father? What would the plan be?" Yes, the thought had crossed our minds, but we never voiced it out loud. Despite some broken bones and periodic sinus infections, my mom was relatively healthy. She visited my dad in the nursing home every day. She was his advocate, partner, and soul mate. She kept him alive through her daily visits and loving attention. It was hard to imagine how we could sustain my father without her.

My brother, sister, and I each had a different answer to my mother's question. "We could move him to Boston, near me," I suggested. "There's actually a pretty good dementia unit not far from my home," my sister offered. My brother, who lived in Michigan at the time, felt my dad should stay put. After considering the pros and cons of a move, we decided that the best option, should our mother die first, was for Dad to stay at the nursing home where he was well cared for and comfortable. My brother, sister, and I would have to come up with a plan to visit Dad regularly and manage his care without my mother. A year after that conversation, my father died. Although the scenario posed by my mother didn't take place, knowing we had agreed upon a plan in case it did lifted a weight off our shoulders.

A mistake that frequently plagues caregivers is not making contingency plans. They rely too heavily on the healthy parent to stay healthy and don't consider alternatives if that scenario should fail. As Steven's father's disease progressed, his mother became the full-time caregiver. To give her a break, Steven hired a home health aide to help out around the house and to bathe and dress his father, who was growing increasingly difficult to handle. Aside from a few bad days when Steven's dad was disoriented and aggressive, the plan seemed to work. Then one day Steven got a call from the hospital. His mother had suffered a stroke.

According to the Alzheimer's Association, a close relationship between a caregiver and care recipient, like spouse or partner, can place the caregiver at higher risk for psychological and physical illness.[4] This is particularly true for "higher hour" caregivers, which the National Alliance for Caregiving defines as providing over twenty-one hours of care per week.[5] Steven's mother provided well over forty hours of care per week. Eventually, Steven's mother was able to return home with the help of paid caregivers who assisted with personal care, laundry, and errands. But she could no longer care for Steven's father. Steven took time off from work so he could cobble together care arrangements for his dad while his mother regained her strength. He worked with the social worker, who identified a memory disorder unit at an assisted living community not far from his mother's home. Steven's father initially resisted the move. When Steven took his father for a dinnertime visit at the facility, the staff was friendly and the atmosphere was welcoming. As luck would have it, Dad's favorite meal of barbecued ribs and mashed potatoes was being served. Steven's father decided that moving to assisted living was not such a bad idea after all. Steven was relieved that he finally had a plan, but regretted that he hadn't been more proactive before his mother's stroke. He may have felt less overwhelmed and perhaps have had more options.

While maintaining a positive outlook is important, one must also be realistic. As a caregiver, sometimes it helps to think like a pessimist. The pessimist may be more inclined to supply a boat with life rafts. That needs to happen before the voyage begins. Dementia is a progressive illness. The parent with Alzheimer's is going to get worse. And the caregiver is eventually going to need help. Steven had not considered the next step—how his mother and father would manage the disease as it progressed. He had not realized there were housing options, such as a continuing care retirement community (CCRC), where his parents could have lived in the same community but with different levels of care. Having more information under his belt might not have changed the outcome, but it would have made the decision-making process less chaotic. Steven focused his attention, as my family did, on the impaired parent, and failed to plan for an alternative scenario in which the caregiving parent gets sick or dies first.

Build a Caregiving Bench—Before a Crisis

The would-have, could-have, should-have lament from caregivers often spills from the same bucket. "I wish I knew what I didn't know and reached out for help sooner," Jane Gross, founding blogger of the *New York Times' New Old Age* blog, writes. She poignantly describes this learn-as-you-go phenomenon in her book *A Bittersweet Season*. Chronicling a trial by fire experience caring for her eighty-five-year-old mother, Gross shares her emotionally wrenching yet ultimately redemptive journey. Through trial, tribulation, and lots of error, Gross traversed the messy landscape of caregiving. She shares valuable information learned en route that she wishes she had known ahead of time, and she offers lessons on what to ask and where to go for answers.

The first place many caregivers go for help is the Internet. According to a Pew Research study, caregivers are more technologically savvy than the rest of the population.[6] Although there are many great resources in the Cloud, googling "caring for aging parents" yields a whopping 1.5 million hits. While some of this information may be useful, the sheer volume of it can be daunting. Gross learned that a trusted guide can help you avoid some of the land mines that dot the landscape of senior care. She ultimately hired a care manager to help her make better decisions about her mother's care. Steven also found that consulting an expert was invaluable. The social worker helped him choose a care facility for his dad and in-home support for his mom. "I only wish I had reached out earlier," he lamented.

Many people just don't know where to go for meaningful and credible help. If you are in the workplace, a good place to start is your employer. We'll go into this topic in more detail in chapter 7. Increasingly, more employers recognize that a growing number of employees are distracted and distressed as a result of caregiving responsibilities. It's hard to pay attention to the year-end financials when you get a call that your mother's caregiver didn't show up. And more companies are realizing the benefits of supporting employees across the life span.

From resources and referrals to temporary backup care, these benefits can mitigate the risks of workday interruptions or bailing out of the workforce entirely.

And then there are the unanticipated costs that are not covered by Medicare, outlined in chapter 5. If you and your family are among the affluent "1 percenters," you are going to have more options for care, although you won't necessarily be spared the grief and guesswork—just the sticker shock. For the rest of you 99 percent, you'll need to figure out how your family member is going to pay for care before you do anything else. That's where elder law attorneys can save you a boatload of time, aggravation, and even money. An elder law attorney specializes in the complex legal and financial issues impacting seniors. Most can handle a wide range of issues such as Medicaid eligibility (which can vary by state), estate planning, and the delegation of healthcare decision making in the event of incompetency. There are about ten thousand lawyers in the United States who specialize in elder law, but how do you find one who is the right fit for your family? While it is best to get a referral from a trusted source, there are websites such as the National Academy of Elder Law Attorneys (www.naela.org) and Elder Law Answers (www.elderlawanswers.com) that provide worthwhile information and a list of elder law attorneys by state.

Long-Distance Caregivers: Where to Turn?

Living a distance from your parents can add another monkey wrench into the mix. While the majority of adult children in the United States live within twenty minutes of their parents, an increasing number of caregivers, like me, live more than an hour away. Long-distance caregiving is a growing global phenomenon. In China, for instance, increased migration from rural to urban areas has exacerbated the caregiver shortage. Transnational caregivers, people who care for elder relatives across national boundaries, have an additional challenge. Stopping by on your way home from work to check on your mother just isn't an option. Many will rely on informal supports, other family members, friends, and neighbors to help out with care-related duties.

Having eyes and ears (other than your own) can be essential to ensuring that family members are getting the help they need. Individuals termed "aging life care professionals" by the Aging Life Care Association (they are also known as care managers) are an invaluable resource, especially for long-distance caregivers. These eldercare experts can be found through the organization's website (www.aginglifecare.org) and are typically social workers, nurses, and other healthcare professionals knowledgeable about local resources and care providers. With skill and finesse, an aging life care professional can connect with your mother and, if all goes well, get her to accept help. Costs range from $100 to $200 per hour, but it's often money well spent. An aging life care professional can steer you in the right direction and save your sanity to boot. If this is beyond your budget, there may be free or low-cost resources worth considering; you just have to know where to look.

In 1965, when life expectancy topped out at seventy-three years old, there was not much of a safety net for older Americans. The period of time between illness and death was relatively short. When my grandfather had a massive stroke and died at seventy-two, it was sad but not unusual. That same year Congress passed the Older Americans Act (OAA) based on a growing concern that seniors did not have easy access to social services, nutrition support, in-home care, and legal assistance. In 1973, amendments to the OAA required states to implement programs and services for older Americans at the local level. The Area Agencies on Aging (also known as AAAs) grew out of this initiative and exist today in a more expanded form. The Area Agencies on Aging are your gateway to local resources and can help you find resources. While these regional support agencies provide much-needed resources for seniors and their caregivers, funding for certain programs may be limited to frail elders who are low income and meet financial eligibility requirements. Information about local providers such as home care agencies, adult day programs, and housing options is free. You may save yourself some grief and guesswork by reaching out to your local Area Agency on Aging through the eldercare locator www.eldercare.gov.

It Takes a Village

Although the Area Agencies on Aging are part of a large nationwide safety net of support, don't overlook informal community-based resources such as friends, neighbors, and religious organizations—a village of sorts. Hillary Rodham Clinton's book *It Takes a Village* promoted the idea that society as a whole can provide a safe and nurturing foundation for families to raise children. The notion that a community can look out for its more vulnerable citizens has great relevance for seniors today, particularly those who are most isolated. Years ago, I had a next-door neighbor, a woman in her late eighties, who lived alone in a large Victorian home she was no longer able to maintain. She was barely able to get in and out during the cold, icy New England winters. A group of concerned neighbors and I got together and checked on her regularly. We made sure she had food, took out her trash, and shoveled her walkway. Eventually a family member stepped in and moved our neighbor to a smaller and hopefully safer setting.

Over the years, I have heard similar heartwarming stories of seniors who relied on the kindness of strangers, neighbors, and friends. Some have found an abundance of goodwill as well as tangible help from local churches, synagogues, mosques, and other religious institutions that seek to support their aging members. Like my neighbor, many of these senior citizens have a strong connection to communities where they've lived most of their lives. And many don't have any intention of moving out, even if their homes are no longer senior-safe.

Consider the Village movement, a growing option for seniors who want to "age in place," staying in their homes and communities. Members of the "Village" pay an annual fee, ranging from $150 to over $500, for access to discount services such as transportation, home modification and repair, in-home care, and meal delivery. Villages don't deliver the services themselves; they work with prescreened providers that offer preferred rates. Since the majority of seniors want to age in place, the Village concept allows them easy access to supports that help them do just that. Go to the Village to Village Network website to find out if there is a village near you: www.vtvnetwork.org.

Learning about different options for care and building a bench may seem like a low priority when your parent is relatively healthy. When you are focused on getting to work, saving for the kids' college, and fixing the broken gutters, life can be a daily and dizzying balancing act. Who has time to anticipate anything that isn't front and center, in your face, demanding immediate attention? Most of us are just trying to get through the day.

When I was pregnant with my first child in the late 1980s, I read *What to Expect When You're Expecting*, a must-read for mothers-to-be at that time. It helped me anticipate the unknown, exciting, and often stressful experience of pregnancy and new motherhood. It focused on life. But what to expect when you're expecting to be a caregiver is a harder pill to swallow. It focuses on the end of life—a voyage we will all travel one day, fraught with frequent and unforeseen forks in the road. My family traveled this winding road for twelve years. Looking back, the abundance of time was a gift. It enabled my family to enter my father's world and continue to hold him close to ours. Whether you assume the mantle of caregiver for years or only months, with some basic knowledge, patience, humor, and compassion, you can prepare yourself for your own unique journey and bare your soul to the inevitable hurt and healing along the way.

TWO

The Imperfect Caregiver

Perfect is the enemy of good.
—VOLTAIRE

One of the greatest challenges of caregiving is the reality that there is no clear path. Twists and turns abound, and no matter how hard you try to get things right, inevitably things go wrong. Caregivers who set an impossibly high standard for themselves (and others) are at the greatest risk of burnout. Personally, I learned about the painful consequences of perfectionism from my daughter, Rebecca. Growing up with two older brothers who set a high bar for achievement, Rebecca—despite her talent, beauty, and smarts—felt she didn't measure up. At age fourteen she developed an eating disorder. Like many young women in the throes of adolescent self-doubt, Rebecca took her anger and frustration out on the most available target—herself. After years of therapy, Rebecca is beginning to quiet the critical voice inside her head and appreciate her own inner beauty and strength. Therapy has helped Rebecca adapt the strategy of "radical acceptance." She is learning to understand what is within her power to change. She also recognizes that anger, guilt, frustration, and sadness are not emotions for which to berate herself, but feelings to gently integrate into an often rocky and unpredictable journey.

Those life lessons of acceptance of what we can and cannot change have great relevance for caregivers. We often expect that our efforts, good intentions, and sheer force of will should shield our loved ones from harm. And sometimes they do. But often, we find ourselves angry at our parents—not to mention ourselves—because things have not gone as planned. The result? Feelings of guilt that we are not doing enough, especially if we fail to convince our parents to accept the help they so desperately need. Why are they making our lives more complicated? And what can we do about it?

Common caregiver frustrations often derive from the

struggle to be a good daughter or son, filial obligations that loom large, contrasted with the reality of parents who don't want help, siblings that don't pitch in, and life demands that keep on coming.

> "My mother sacrificed a great deal to raise me and my siblings. Now it's my turn to take care of her. But between kids, work, and Mom's declining health, I feel resentful that it's all on me."

> "I have tried everything to get Mom to accept help. She fires the caregivers because she doesn't think she needs them. But my mother fell last week carrying the laundry basket and I am really worried."

> "My father would never let a stranger in his home. He is so mistrustful. I am always the one to take him to the doctor, give him his meds, do the grocery shopping, and . . . fill in the blank."

Sound familiar? Join the club. At times you may feel isolated, overburdened, and ineffective. You'll lament the disconnect between your efforts and actual outcomes. You may feel like the mythological Greek king Sisyphus, condemned in Hades to endlessly push an immense boulder to the top of a hill, only to have it roll back down each time. Sometimes you need to step away from the boulder to realize that you are pushing in the wrong direction.

Be Okay with Good Enough

It took Barbara a trip to the emergency room with what she thought was a heart attack to change course and adopt a more self-compassionate approach to caregiving. Barbara was a professional caregiver—a pediatric nurse in her late forties, married with two adolescent sons. Friends compared her to Martha Stewart, exacting in her attention to even the smallest details of domestic life. Barbara was one of those people about whom everyone said, "I don't know how she does it." While proud of her life and accomplishments, Barbara felt exhausted and uninspired most of the time. This in turn made her feel guilty and resentful.

Barbara's oldest son, Ben, was a high school basketball star and an all-around good kid. He had been awarded a full scholarship to a state university close to home and was going to graduate with honors in the spring. Alex, the younger son, was a different story. Diagnosed with learning disabilities in middle school, Alex suffered from low self-esteem and was often belligerent and distant. Now a freshman in high school, Alex behaved like a typical teenager—dirty clothes strewn across his room, ear buds perpetually attached to his head, and monosyllabic responses to Barbara's seemingly innocuous inquiries about his day. Afraid of pushing Alex further away, Barbara backed off on her expectations. Alex hardly ever remembered to take out the trash, shovel the driveway, or walk the dog. To add to the tension, Barbara and her husband Ralph often fought over how best to handle Alex.

While Barbara loved her job on an inpatient pediatric unit, she typically cared for children with life-threatening diseases, and it took an emotional toll. Barbara's secret fantasy was to check in to a hotel room, order room service, watch reruns of *The Bachelorette*, and not talk to anyone! She would muse about this guilty pleasure as she ran her errands after work. After making a multicourse dinner, she would catch up on emails and bills, then collapse. There was little room in her life for an eldercare crisis.

When Barbara first got the call that her eighty-two-year-old mother had had a stroke, she was upset but optimistic. Barbara's mother was fiercely independent—some would say stubborn. Barbara assumed that her mother would recover and, after a stint in rehab, return to a life of independence. The initial few weeks of hospitalization and rehabilitation were agonizing. Barbara's mother failed to make progress and doctors suggested she consider a nursing home. "Are you kidding?" Barbara exclaimed. "Out of the question!" Barbara had vowed never to put her mother in a nursing home, but clearly she could not return home alone. So Barbara cleared out Ben's room, ordered a hospital bed, and set things up for Mom to stay with her—at least temporarily. Since Barbara was a nurse, she anticipated that caring for Mom would be challenging but manageable. Barbara hired a home health aide to care for her mother during the day and put herself "on duty" the moment she walked in the front door.

Within weeks, things began to unravel. The home health aide could not get Barbara's mom out of bed. Alex was of little help and frequently complained that their home had turned into a makeshift hospital. Ralph had taken on a new contracting job and, though sympathetic to Barbara's situation, he was unable to pitch in as much as she would have liked. Worst of all, Barbara's mother was unhappy. She did not like having so little control over her life and took her frustration out on Barbara. Just as things seemed like they could not get any harder, the home health aide quit. That's when Barbara began to feel the heart palpitations.

Not until she was in the emergency room and the attending doctor ordered a psychiatric consult did Barbara recognize that her situation was unsustainable. The good news was that she had not had a heart attack. The bad news was that her anxiety was so severe it felt like one. Barbara began to examine the boulders she was pushing. She realized she had set unrealistic expectations for herself. She could not be everyone's caregiver at home and simultaneously maintain a full-time demanding job that required a high level of compassion and skill. She was neglecting her own needs. The caregiving reservoir was being depleted. But Barbara still felt stuck. Because she was a nurse, she felt she had to be the one among her siblings to oversee her mother's care.

Fortunately, she realized that overseeing didn't mean she actually had to do everything. Barbara organized a family meeting and created a list of tasks she had previously assumed herself. She made an agenda. She told her siblings there was a lot at stake—not just their mother's health, but her own. Barbara's brother agreed to pitch in to help manage Mom's finances and any legal work that needed to be done. Barbara's sister offered to research options for care. Eventually the siblings presented Barbara's mother with a plan—sell her house and move to an assisted living community. Initially resistant to the idea, Barbara's mother balked. But with encouragement from her children and the healthcare team, she came to recognize that remaining at home would be unsafe. And the senior community seemed nice enough. There were meals every day, activities for the residents, and even an on-site hairdresser.

After the move, Barbara visited her mother several

times a week and was surprised to see how well she was adjusting to the new surroundings. She even made a new friend, a recently widowed woman who shared her passion for opera (which was telecast from the Met for the residents to enjoy). While the effects of the stroke were considerable, Barbara's mother regained enough function to manage daily activities with the help of an occasional caregiver.

Barbara's trip to the emergency room brought about some other needed changes. She paid more attention to her body and the way she reacted to stress. She examined her perfectionism and began accepting her own limitations. She came to understand that her desire to be perfect was an unhealthy form of self-validation. It was how she proved to herself that she was a caring person worthy of love. But it also exacted a price and made her angry, overwhelmed, and resentful. So rather than simply pile more things onto her already overloaded plate, Barbara began to judiciously pare down her "to do" list and delegate to others.

As a result, she had more time to devote to Alex, giving him the attention he needed but pushed away. Barbara even persuaded Alex to come along on visits to the assisted living community. To Barbara's surprise, Alex developed a remarkable ability to engage with his grandmother, shucking with her the surly adolescent veneer he donned with his own parents.

Of course, Barbara's life was still stressful. She and her husband occasionally fought about Alex's challenging behavior—just less often. She still got the occasional phone call that her mother was unhappy about X, Y, or Z. But Barbara stopped rushing in to save the day. She enlisted the support of her siblings. She worked with the staff at the assisted living community and tried to address problems before they mushroomed into a crisis. Gradually, she let go of her own need to be the perfect mother, wife, and daughter—which wasn't working anyway. Barbara lowered her standards of making home-cooked meals during the week and stopped for takeout more often. One fateful evening, she assigned dinner preparation to Alex and Ralph. The pasta tasted like mush and the salad was wilted. But for Barbara the ability to let go was something to savor, bringing with it a newfound sense of freedom.

Years later Barbara's mom had a second stroke. This one was far more debilitating and the assisted living community could no longer manage her care. With great difficulty, the family made the decision to move Barbara's mother to a nearby nursing home. The building was old and tired, but the nurses and aides were patient and attentive, so that was good enough. Barbara realized that her "vow" to never put her mother in a nursing home had been made in a vacuum, without knowledge or experience.

Barbara cherished visits with her mom, who was still able to recognize her daughter and express some measure of affection—although in a subtle, slightly backhanded way. On one visit, Barbara brought an old photo album of her tenth birthday party. Barbara, in a pixie haircut, was smiling ear to ear, surrounded by girlfriends and presents. "Look, Mom!" Barbara said. "You baked your famous Boston cream pie birthday cake. Do you remember that day?" Barbara's mom hesitated for a moment, pointed to the photo, and said, "I never liked that haircut." Barbara smiled and hugged her mother. "Neither did I," she said.

The caregiving experience taught Barbara many things. She learned to be more open to change to best accommodate reality. She became more forgiving of herself and others and more appreciative of the most important relationships in her life. And she was able to recognize that although these relationships were highly imperfect, they were, nonetheless, immeasurably precious.

Lessons Learned: You Can't Do It All

Although this statement may seem obvious, caregivers are often like the proverbial frog in hot water. If you drop a frog into hot water, so the story goes, it will immediately jump out. But if you put a frog in cool water and gradually increase the temperature, the frog adjusts, stays where it is, and eventually boils. Many caregivers are oblivious to their deteriorating health and well-being as they pile more and more onto their overloaded plates. Like many sandwich-generation caregivers caught between the needs of their parents and children, Barbara was slowly getting boiled. And as in Barbara's experience, it often takes a crisis to jolt people out of this pattern. But knowing the risks *ahead of time* can potentially prevent problems from spiraling out of control.

Manage Expectations, Including Yours

One of the greatest risks for caregivers is that expectations of themselves and others can be unattainably high. My father had numerous caregivers in the nursing home. Some were excellent; others were mediocre. We learned to work with the team as it was, encouraging the positive. We did address problems with staff and quality of care, but only when it was important—like failing to properly treat a urinary tract infection. On the other hand, when someone once dressed Dad in another resident's trousers, it was an innocuous mistake we chose to ignore. Barbara started off like many caregivers, thinking that she could do it all and do it better than anyone else. She was quickly disabused of this notion and needed to adjust her expectations—starting with her own fallibility. This is particularly hard for people in caregiving professions like Barbara, who are used to being the one relied upon, not the one who needs to accept help from others.

Be Adaptable

Many, if not most of us, tend to overschedule our lives (and our children's); we make plans and then execute them. With caregiving, often your best-conceived plans morph into something very different down the road. Prepare to make adjustments quickly. When Barbara's plan A failed, she tried plan B—the assisted living option. And when that was no longer viable, Barbara came up with plan C, the nursing home. It helps to consider these options ahead of time, discuss "what-ifs" with family, so you can more nimbly make decisions as the situation changes.

Don't Make Promises You Can't—or Shouldn't—Keep

"Never say never!" a friend once said. She had sworn off ever buying her child toy guns when she was pregnant. "But he really wanted it!" she explained after she bought her four-year-old son a Nerf gun. Most of us start our caregiving journey with strong prescriptions about what we will and will not do. Ask any mom or dad if they stayed true to their ideal of parenting and you will get a resounding *no* from the honest ones. Stupid mom and stupid dad stories have become an amusing and accepted part of our national conversation—even a rite of passage. But stupid adult daughter stories? Or guilt-ridden son stories? Not so much. And when you bring up the unspeakable— nursing home—people really start to make judgments, however unspoken. I still feel the need to explain that my mother was unable to handle my father's care and that he was much better off in a nursing home. But many people, like Barbara, make pronouncements about how they will handle a parent's care before they have any idea what type of care may be needed. Making informed decisions based on needs as they *evolve* may avoid the perils that Barbara faced and pave the way for safer and more suitable care.

Get Help

This advice is so much trickier than it seems. Where do you start? Your brother? What will he offer? Criticism, advice, and then . . . silence. Your sister? After she exploded at you for not remembering her anniversary? Seriously? You can barely remember your own anniversary! Even if your siblings can offer only limited support, most of the time it is better than nothing. At least they will be in the loop.

What about those harried doctors? And the nurses in the hospital who seem to be wearing roller skates. They barely have time to say hello, never mind give you an update. Communicating with medical professionals requires effort, but it will help you better advocate for your parents and understand their medical status.

If you need more in-home help, consider hiring a professional caregiver through a local home care agency or a website such as Care.com. Some families build in respite care to get temporary relief from the day-to-day responsibilities of caregiving. Respite care can be provided by a paid caregiver, volunteer, or senior community such as an assisted living facility. For information on respite care resources nationwide, go to the National Respite Locator Service at www.archrespite.org. Making sure you get a break from time to time will help you go the distance and avoid caregiver burnout.

Barbara eventually realized she couldn't do it all and had to get better at accepting help. She came to embrace being a caregiver while at the same time acknowledging her own needs. She knew she was not perfect and learned to be okay with good enough. And so did Barbara's mom. Despite initial resistance, she eventually accepted help and stopped relying solely on Barbara.

Some families never get to this point and remain stuck in the struggle. So what do you do when your parent flat-out refuses help? This all too common phenomenon is like the quicksand of senior care. You step in, get dragged down, and need to find a way out somehow.

THREE

The Parent Who Rejects Help

You cannot save people, you can only love them.
—ANAÏS NIN

No matter how impaired or intransigent our mothers and fathers may be, they are still our parents. We inadvertently infantilize our parents and deputize ourselves when we suggest that caregiving is a role reversal. But it is a profound life-altering shift of roles that requires balancing the right to self-determination with the recognition that your parents need help. And sometimes they won't find that balance on their own. How do you respect your mother's autonomy when she insists on cooking even though she can't be trusted with the stove? What do you do when your father is cleaning gutters just months after knee surgery (and your mom is holding the ladder)? And how do you stay sane when a crisis is just one phone call away? One of the biggest frustrations for adult children is that they come up with a plan that makes perfect sense to them but their parent says, "Thanks but no thanks." How hard do you push? When do you back away?

Years ago at a talk I was giving on help-rejecting parents, Catherine, an elegant woman with well-coifed hair and a poised matter-of-fact manner, shared her story. Catherine's parents were staunch Republicans living in northern Maine—an isolated area with few people and lots of snow. Her father, in his late eighties, continued to shovel his walkway and roof. Catherine pleaded with him to get help before he suffered an injury—or worse. He stubbornly refused, insisting he was perfectly fine on his own. At wit's end, Catherine hatched a plan. Every month she told her father she would deposit money into an account earmarked for snow removal only. If by July the money was still there, it would be donated to the Democratic National Committee. I never found out if Catherine's plan worked, but I marveled at her ability to use humor and creativity to get through a caregiving impasse.

When our parents' refusal to accept help puts their safety and well-being in jeopardy, we feel compelled to act, yet our good intentions are often thwarted. Catherine could not stop her father from shoveling snow, but she could try strategic persuasion to alter his behavior. Over the years, I have heard countless stories of caregivers who tried strong-arming their parent to accept help—only to feel angry and dismayed when their efforts failed. As we look after our aging parents, we do so with a mixture of love, devotion, and a desire to care for the person who sacrificed so much to care for us. When it's time to hire outside help, we may experience a mixture of relief and regret. As my father's dementia worsened, he made it easy on us. When we hired caregivers, he greeted them with his trademark smile, which lessened our guilt and grief. But for other good sons and daughters, getting your parent to accept help may require more than just strategy, patience, and a plan. It may take a crisis. In Chinese, the word for crisis has two characters. One for danger—the other for opportunity. As a parent's decline progresses, resistance may erode too. A window of opportunity may open as your parent is more amenable to help—hopefully before it is too late.

Home Alone

Like many mothers and daughters, Rachel and her mother Sally had a close and tempestuous relationship. Although tensions had subsided over the years, old conflicts re-surfaced as Rachel pushed her mom to face facts. At eighty-eight, Sally was losing ground. Rachel insisted her mother wasn't safe in the home where she'd lived for fifty years. Rachel looked into retirement communities that had units all on one floor with senior-safe showers and tubs. But Sally wouldn't budge. Her home was a warm, familiar place—filled with memories of her children and husband Lenny, who had passed away years earlier, leaving Sally bereft and alone. Sally had relied on Lenny for many things: paying bills, maintaining the house, taking care of the cars, and driving.

Few aspects of senior care are more combustible and conflict-ridden than the big D: driving. The idea that your mother, who can barely see or hear her television, takes control of a four-thousand-pound machine to tootle around town—well, that might keep you up at night. And you may have reason to worry. Per mile traveled, fatal crashes increase significantly starting at ages seventy to seventy-four and are highest among drivers eighty-five and older.[1] Although older drivers as a group are generally safe, they have a higher risk of injury or death if they do get in an accident because they are less likely to be able to withstand physical trauma. Just because your mom is eighty-five doesn't necessarily mean she should stop driving. My mother is eighty-eight and continues to make the two-hour drive to visit my family on a regular basis. But she knows her limits and modifies her driving accordingly. She avoids the high-speed lane, doesn't drive at night, obeys the speed limit and, like UPS, 90 percent of the time doesn't take left-hand turns.[2]

Years ago when my father started getting lost in familiar places, we worried that it was time to hand over the keys. Massachusetts General Hospital psychiatrist Dr. William Falk delivered the tough message. On a prescription pad, he wrote his recommendation that my father no longer drive, and gently gave it to my dad. This symbolic gesture felt absolute and unwavering. As painful as it was, the message was received and accepted. Of all the losses my father suffered during those early years of dementia, this was perhaps the greatest blow. Giving up driving can feel like a bereavement. It is a profound loss of independence that often heralds a cascade of losses to come.

While my father gave up driving without a fight, Sally insisted she was safe behind the wheel despite evidence to the contrary. And Rachel was worried. She questioned the numerous dings and dents on Sally's newly leased car. "Someone must have hit my car in the supermarket parking lot," Sally explained. Rachel wasn't buying it. Rachel's impulse was to take the keys away, but she knew her mother would be resistant and find a way to drive anyway. So rather than presenting Sally with a fait accompli, Rachel sparked a conversation with questions expressing her genuine concern and interest.

"How would you get around if you couldn't drive anymore?"

"Are you limiting driving at all?"

"Are there times you feel anxious behind the wheel?"

"Would there be a benefit to not driving at all, such as no auto insurance and no car maintenance and repairs?"

Rachel eventually got her mother to agree to a driving assessment and hired an instructor who worked with seniors and disabled adults. Not since her own road test thirty years earlier had Rachel been so anxious in a car. As she sat white-knuckled in the back seat, Rachel observed her mother making excuses for missed turn signals and erratic lane changes. "I'm not used to this car," Sally explained. The instructor (who had full control over the vehicle) was patient, respectful, and firm. When he told Sally she had flunked the road test, Rachel was relieved. Sally was angry, upset, and bereaved.

While Sally ultimately stopped driving, many people

who participate in evaluations can continue to drive safely. They may receive recommendations on improving their skills, avoiding certain conditions, or adapting equipment to make driving safer. There are numerous steps you can and should take before taking the keys away. The American Automobile Association (AAA) provides detailed information on the different types of driving evaluations and their associated costs.[3] The AARP driver safety program focuses on mobility, technology, and driver safety for older adults.[4] ChORUS (the Clearinghouse for Older Road User Safety) is a great resource for information pertaining to highway safety for aging drivers. But despite your best efforts, there may come a time when your parent has to hang up the keys.

When Sally had to stop driving she was devastated, but she was also willing to consider outside help. And *there* was the opening. Rachel persuaded her mother to hire a professional caregiver, who assumed the roles of chauffeur, housekeeper, and companion. Rachel breathed a sigh of relief.

While the caregiver was helpful, Sally was still alone for a good part of each day. She was becoming more confused and less able to manage even small things on her own. So Rachel convinced Sally to wear a Life Alert bracelet that automatically calls for help if it detects a fall. It's a wonderful piece of technology that can be a lifesaver—but only if you wear it.

It was a frigid winter day and Sally's caregiver Meghan had just finished her six-hour shift and headed home. Sally had begrudgingly accepted Meghan, a no-nonsense woman in her mid-forties who was both competent and kind. Although she did not often admit it, Sally looked forward to Meghan's company and had grown to rely on her. But Sally also treasured her time alone at the end of the day when she could watch TV or read a book in solitude. After Meghan left, Sally decided to make a cup of tea as she watched the evening news—her nightly ritual. As Sally threw away the tea bag, she noticed the garbage bin was getting full. Always a fastidious homemaker (Rachel would say OCD), Sally decided she would take out the garbage herself. Wearing only a thin wool sweater, cotton slacks, and slippers, Sally descended the stairs to the garage. And then it happened. Sally missed a step, tripped, and fell. Alone in the dark, without a cell phone or her emergency alert bracelet (left on the nightstand), Sally panicked. She yelled for help but no one could hear her. She tried in vain to push herself back up the stairs into the warmth of her home. But she was frozen in place. Then Sally felt an agonizing pain as the cold damp air stung her face and filled her lungs.

Rachel was on vacation with her husband and ten-year-old son when she got the call from Meghan. Rachel could almost hear Meghan's heart race as she recounted her story. Meghan had arrived at Sally's home at 9:30 a.m., her usual time. When she saw the newspaper on the front step, she worried something was amiss. Sally usually got out of bed by 8 a.m., made herself toast and coffee, and read the paper or watched TV. Typically when Meghan walked in the front door, she heard the television blaring at an ear-piercing volume. But as Meghan entered Sally's house that day, she was greeted by stark silence and an eerie stillness. Meghan ran to the bedroom and saw the bed had not been slept in. She checked the bathroom, but there was no sign of Sally. She called Sally's name, but there was no response. Meghan was nearly panicking, imagining the worst. After an exhaustive search of the house, she opened the door to the garage and heard a barely audible moan. There was Sally—her eyes bulging with pain and fear, her breathing shallow and labored. Meghan called 911, laid a blanket over Sally, and prayed.

After a long, terrifying night in the cold garage, Sally's temperature had fallen to eighty-six degrees. She was experiencing hypothermia—a dangerous drop in body temperature caused by prolonged exposure to the cold. Sally had been in excruciating pain, having suffered a fractured hip compounded by a night lying sprawled on the garage floor. The doctors said that if Meghan hadn't arrived when she did, Sally would not have survived much longer.

Rachel cut her vacation short and rushed back home. The restful calm of a few days' vacation was replaced by a morbid dread. Would her mom survive? Would she ever walk again? What type of care would she need—or accept? After surgery and a short hospital stay, Sally was transferred to a rehab facility, where she recuperated for two months. At first Sally was slow to cooperate, but the physical therapists were skilled and eventually helped Sally overcome her fears. Gradually she regained the ability to walk, first with a walker, then a cane. She returned home and agreed to 24/7 in-home care—an expensive alternative to nursing home care that the family was fortunate to be able to afford. Although Sally became incontinent and increasingly more confused, she was surprisingly content. Rachel, after battling with her mother to accept help for years, could finally stop fighting. "I never thought Mom would come home again and be able to walk," she says. "She fought everything. Now she is more accepting and less anxious. I am less overwhelmed. My mother is in good hands and seems happy to be taken care of. And I am grateful she is still here."

Years ago, when I was the director of discharge planning at a community hospital, I saw firsthand what happens when at-risk frail elders refuse help. Sooner or later, like Sally, they fall, confuse medications, get sick, or injure themselves. If they end up in the hospital, discharge options may be limited and time frames tight. Families are given short notice to make important long-term care decisions in the midst of a crisis. For folks like Sally, a crisis may precipitate change. But unlike Sally, few people have the financial resources to pay for around-the-clock care.

Sally was also fortunate to have a devoted daughter who realized her mother's headstrong attitude could also be a strength. After all, Sally's determination and tenacity helped her survive a long cold night in the garage with a broken hip. And to Rachel's surprise, Sally eventually was able to accept help and trust a stranger who became both caregiver and friend—and who ultimately saved her life. "My mother continued to grow and evolve, even with dementia and disabilities," Rachel mused. "Who knows what challenges and opportunities old age will bring?"

A Difficult Balance

Erik Erikson, an internationally renowned child psychoanalyst, identified eight stages of human development, each with a discrete challenge and opportunity, that a healthy person traverses over the course of a lifetime.[5]

The infant who bonds with a loving parent achieves basic trust. The young adult seeks intimacy and risks isolation. And the senior feels contentment for what has been achieved or despair for what has not. The challenge of each life stage can be accepted and embraced, allowing us to integrate our emotional polarity and achieve wisdom and understanding.

Erikson's wife and collaborator, Joan Erikson, added a ninth stage for the eighty-five-plus cohort, now the fastest-growing demographic in the United States.[6] In this final stage, which Erikson called the woven cycle of life, previous threads of development are revisited and the risk of mistrust and despair looms large. As elders lose their capacity to care for themselves, they become more vulnerable to shame and self-doubt. Yet hope can be restored. Trust can be achieved. And through empathy and love, despair can be averted.

So, is the message that if we love our parents enough they will accept help? No. Probably not. But we *can* strive to accept our parents' limitations—and our own. We can interpret their stubbornness, like Sally's, as a fear of loss of control. We can work with them—as much as possible—and not against them. We can empathize with their fears and not take their resistance personally. But that doesn't mean we accept any behavior, no matter how problematic and risky, and allow ourselves to be whipsawed and trodden upon, like a caregiving doormat.

It's a difficult balance: trying to support our parents' right to make independent decisions that may put them at risk while protecting them from their own bad choices. We may coax, cajole, and humor our elders into accepting help. But we may ultimately need to back off. We also need to be aware when we are putting our own well-being and health at risk.

The Daughter Trap

"I've got daughters. So I don't need more help," explained Ed, a strong-willed eighty-five-year-old with type 2 diabetes that was spiraling out of control. "He's got a hardheaded thing going on," Jan said of her stepfather. "But he raised me since I was a toddler after my biological father walked out. He's a cool guy and a wonderful dad." In the months after Jan's mother died, Ed's health markedly declined. Ed grew more confused, driving around not knowing where he was and frequently forgetting to take his insulin. When his blood sugar spiked to a dangerous degree, Ed refused to go the hospital. Jan, upset and alarmed, pleaded with her stepfather and eventually called 911 against his wishes.

Diabetes can be a tough disease to manage. Adherence

to a daily regimen of medication, diet, and medical monitoring requires constant vigilance and can lead to noncompliance.[7] Families typically provide the lion's share of care to loved ones like Ed, who often don't make it easy. Since Jan was unmarried, she was the daughter designated to take it all on. Her sisters were too busy with jobs and kids to be much help. As an African American, Jan felt bound by duty, devotion, and cultural expectations. "We don't put our family members in nursing homes if we can take care of them ourselves," she said.

Money was also a worry. Funds were scarce and Ed insisted on paying bills, bouncing a few checks in the process. After leaving her temp job to be a full-time caretaker, Jan could no longer afford her apartment. So Jan moved in with Ed and braced herself for the rough road ahead. Jan had barely unpacked her boxes before things really went south.

First Ed spent a week in the hospital and had two toes amputated. Then he was discharged home with infected ulcers. Exhausted and overwhelmed, Jan felt she had to be both nurse and nanny. She changed Ed's medication-infused bandages, cooked, cleaned, and drove him to medical appointments. But despite all her efforts, the ulcers worsened and Ed's leg had to be amputated. Although Ed was able to put on his own prosthetic, he refused to do so and was confined to a wheelchair. Compounding things further, Ed would not agree to an outdoor ramp, making movement in and out of the house a Herculean task. He was stuck—physically and emotionally. And so was Jan.

Jan could not remember when she last got her hair cut, went to the gym, had lunch with a friend, or simply took time for herself. And like many caregivers, Jan was ignoring her own health—despite the fact that she was feeling sad and sluggish. The wake-up call came from an unexpected source—Ed himself. Ed began to worry about Jan's health and urged her to see a doctor. When Jan finally did, it was bad news. Jan too was diabetic. It was time to get more help and learn to say no.

"I can't do this on my own any longer." Jan said to her sister. Rather than ask tentatively as she had done in the past, Jan explained matter-of-factly what she needed: help on evenings and weekends with their father's care. Then Jan told Ed he didn't have the choice to refuse the ramp— it was going to happen. Jan even found grant funding through the city department of planning to pay for the ramp installation. Next Jan took control of the finances and set up online accounts. "When I showed him the bank balance each month he relaxed and let me take charge," Jan explained. "And when I was able to wheel him in and out of the house, he was happy about the ramp! I even got him to put on his prosthetic so he wouldn't be stuck in the wheelchair all day. I learned I could not always wait for my father to agree to everything. Sometimes I just had to go ahead and do stuff. And the funny thing was—Dad was okay with that."

In the face of strong parental resistance, many adult children, like Jan, either give in, give up, or get angry. While feelings of frustration and anger are a normal part of caregiving, they need a safe outlet. When there isn't one, caregivers may turn on themselves or their loved ones. In extreme cases, a caregiver can become abusive or neglectful, putting a parent's safety at risk. But more often, good daughters and sons become victims of their own inability to set limits and reset expectations. So how can you get your parents to accept the help they need—but don't necessarily want?

Reframe Resistance

"Old age ain't no place for sissies." Bette Davis's famous quote doesn't sugarcoat growing old. Age chips away at our memory, eyesight, hearing, and stamina, and our mobility can slow down along with our metabolisms. As the years roll on, we may be more likely to resemble Mama Cass than the forever-fit Jane Fonda. It's not all bad news, though. People who have healthy lifestyles, eat well, exercise regularly, and enjoy positive social relationships are more likely to enjoy an active and vibrant old age. And they may have more time and space in their life to appreciate the good stuff.

But for many, the twilight years are not necessarily an oasis of good health. More than a quarter of all Americans and two out of three older ones suffer from multiple chronic illnesses.[8] That could make anyone feel vulnerable, afraid, and a bit cranky. Our parents, especially those with chronic illnesses, may fear losing their independence and reject help as a means of exerting control. If we understand resistance as a way to "take arms against a sea of troubles," then we can accept there may be pros and cons to our parents' stubbornness. The "I'll do it my way" approach that put Sally at risk may also have been part of a survival instinct that kept her alive in the cold garage. If we offer ultimatums to our parents, we may find ourselves making empty threats and fighting losing battles. But if we practice empathy, toward our parents and ourselves, we may come up with a workable plan without sacrificing our sanity. We may surrender the battle but ultimately win the war.

Start Small and Offer Options

The idea that a crisis may prompt our parent to ultimately accept help is a grim reality for some, like Rachel and her mother Sally. But offering choices and ceding a little control along the way may help break down walls of resistance. If your mother needs a caregiver, include her in the hiring process. If you're concerned about driving, discuss alternative means of transportation. If your father refuses to leave his home, look into the feasibility and costs of home modification. Sometimes less is more. Pushing too much help too soon can backfire and build more barriers. Hiring a stranger to help a senior get dressed can feel like an indignity. Xenophobia may kick in and your mother may find all kinds of reasons why she doesn't like the caregiver.

Sometimes an indirect approach is better than a frontal assault. For example, the Bourne family's solution to their father's resistance was to lose the term *caregiver*. Cliff Bourne had dementia and was getting to the point where he needed—but adamantly refused—a paid caregiver. A retired CEO, Cliff was used to being in charge and not accustomed to relinquishing control. But when he urinated in the closet instead of the bathroom, his kids knew they had to act. So they came up with the idea of hiring a part-time "assistant." The assistant would prepare meals, take Cliff on walks, do a little laundry, and help out around the house. Over time, the assistant won Cliff's trust and was able to increase her hours and perform personal care-related tasks with skill and compassion.

Recruit Outsiders

One of the golden rules of caregiving is *Don't go it alone.* Like Jan, we often take on more than we can handle rather than persuade our parents to accept help. But if your parent rejects commonsense solutions, stop preaching from a lone bully pulpit and get yourself a Greek chorus. Whom should you recruit? The doctor might convince your grandmother that driving with dementia is not a good idea. Or your brother can take the lead for a change. Trusted neighbors may be willing to help out with errands and food shopping. Or Aunt Alice may be the best one to persuade your mother to move. If, despite your best efforts, your parent won't budge, you may need professional help. Aging life care professionals, elder law attorneys, and professional mediators can provide an objective perspective about financial and legal matters and lay out options for care. They may also dislodge entrenched parents from unreasonable and unsustainable positions that put themselves and others at risk.

Accept Your Limits

Tune into your body. Is your head pounding, stomach churning, back aching? Do you resent doing so much yet feel guilty it's not enough? Recognize that you can't be wonder woman (or man). You have limits and your parents do too. If your father's gruff personality resembles Clint Eastwood's, don't expect kindly Mr. Rogers. Or your Mother Teresa–modeled mom may take care of everyone else but refuse help from others. You can't change them. Your parents have the right to make their own decisions— even bad ones. But you love them anyway.

When All Else Fails

Those caring for a parent with dementia know that the gradual ebbing away of physical and mental capacities can be agonizing. Short-term memory, driving, toileting, and personal hygiene are all causalities in a battle that has no victor—only victims. Watching my remarkably intelligent father lose so many of his abilities was devastating. But our grief was lessened by my father's good-natured acceptance of his own condition. When my mother once scolded my dad, who was supposed to be on a heart-smart diet, for eating greasy potato chips, he smiled and replied, "What do you want from me? I'm senile!"

Eventually it came time for my mother to assume guardianship, a crucial legal tool that allows one person to make decisions on behalf of another who is considered to be incapacitated. We explained this to my father as best we could. He didn't fight us. He trusted we'd make the right choices and take good care of him. Many families are thrown into agonizing struggles with parents whose mental capacities are profoundly impaired. To take away individual rights through the guardianship process, your parent must be more than just stubborn and unreasonable. Your parent, like my father, must be deemed incapacitated by a physician and a judge must agree. A guardian, also known as a conservator, becomes the legal representative who can make financial, medical, and care-related decisions on your parent's behalf. Determining that a parent requires guardianship is a high bar—as it should be. For families like mine, it painfully highlights the truth. Your parent is no longer in the driver's seat and may have to rely on you or another family member to steer the right course.

Most families will never need to take this step. For Rachel and Jan, who each tried persuading her parent to accept help, things eventually had to get worse before they got better. But getting a parent to accept help is just half the battle. What if your sister insists nothing is wrong when your mother is failing right before your eyes? Or your brother exerts control but refuses to pitch in? What if no one is in charge and everyone is at odds? That's what makes this stuff so hard. Your family, for better and worse, is in this together. Somehow, despite bickering and smoldering resentments, you must find common ground—not just with your parents, but your siblings too.

FOUR

Good, Bad, and Nonexistent Siblings

Siblings: Children of the same parents, each of whom is
perfectly normal until they get together.
—SAM LEVENSON

I still remember the look on my mom's face when she
walked into the living room, alarmed by the loud thwack.
It was the sound of a jar being hurled across the room and
smashed against the wall. There were shattered shards of
broken glass everywhere. I was about nine years old—
standing red faced, indignant, ready to plead my case. My
seven-year-old brother was wailing. To this day, I don't
remember what he did to provoke me. I was usually a
pretty easygoing kid—despite the occasional act of violence against my brother. It seemed that every once in a

while, our close, playful relationship would turn sour. And when it did, sparks—or a glass jar—would start to fly.

Sibling conflict is as old as humanity. I imagine little cave brothers and sisters fighting over cave Mommy and Daddy's attention. The Bible's cautionary tale of sibling rivalry gone overboard led to the first murder, that of Abel by his brother Cain. Then there's Joseph, whose jealous brothers stole his multicolored coat and sold him to the Ishmaelites. While our ancient ancestors had a lot of challenges to contend with, at least life was simpler then—because most of them were dead before the age of forty! And their parents were long gone too. Most likely, they were more worried about the saber-toothed tiger than whether Mom should be in a nursing home.

Over the years, I've had my share of sibling squabbles. As the middle child, I was sandwiched between a high-achieving older sister and an adored kid brother. There were rivalries and resentments and a few memorable outbursts. Years after the jar incident, I smashed a blow dryer over my brother's head. His skull survived. (The blow dryer—not so much.) In an excerpt from my diary (June 1969), I describe my brother as a moron and my sister as a blockhead. It's hard to believe, given these insults and injuries, that we grew up to have close, loving relationships as adults.

As my brother, sister, and I grew up and did our best to mature, sibling rivalries subsided and connections deepened. We supported each other through parenting, divorce, cancer, and the gradual and ultimate loss of our father. During the course of my father's illness, there were many decisions to be made and tasks to be undertaken. When my father died, my sister and I supported my mother through the funeral arrangements and my brother handled the avalanche of paperwork that followed. We were more fortunate than many. As we grew into adulthood, my siblings and I had a foundation of trust and communication that served us well when making decisions about my father's care.

But that is not the case for many people. All too often, even deep bonds between siblings can be fractured by the emotionally wrenching experience of caring for an aging parent. For the growing number of adults who find themselves in a blended family, with stepparents and stepsiblings, there's no lifelong foundation to fall back on. Stepbrothers and stepsisters may barely know—or even like—one another. The generation most likely to have stepchildren, the baby boomers, will soon be needing care, and not everyone gets along like the kids in *The Brady Bunch*. It's hard enough to work things out with your own family, but having stepsiblings may add to the number of conflicting opinions. Money can also lead to disagreements. What if your father starts to decline and your stepmother controls the purse strings (and her children are concerned about their inheritance)? Having good relationships with your father's spouse will help, but may not prevent struggles among the adult children. Figuring out how to divvy up caregiving duties can be particularly challenging for blended families, especially if relationships are tenuous to begin with and responsibilities blurred.

The Juggling Act

One of the big hurdles for siblings is the tendency to cling to an ideal of fairness—perhaps an attempt to correct perceived childhood inequities. Yet the burden of caregiving is seldom divvied up equally, like pieces of a pie. Instead, one child, more often a daughter, is saddled with the lion's share of responsibility. Sixty percent of family caregivers are female.[1] The role of the primary caregiver most often falls to women, but men are caregivers too and may also take on more than they can manage. Most family caregivers do their best to juggle it all, but it takes skill, patience, and a willingness to let a few balls drop now and then to make it all work.

When I was a sophomore at Tufts University, I took a

course in human cognitive development from Anita Olds, a pioneer in early childhood architecture and design who held a doctorate in human development and social psychology from Harvard University. Professor Olds decided that her students should compare cognitive theories of development to a real-life experience by learning how to juggle. So I bought the book *Juggling for Klutzes*, a precursor to the "Fill-in-the-Blank for Dummies" series. By the end of the course I was hooked. At the height of my skill, I could do the reverse three-ball cascade and the four-ball fountain. But I really didn't learn how to juggle *life* until I became a caregiver. Like many caregivers, I had a lot of balls in the air—three kids, a full-time job, a traveling spouse, and a father with dementia. Like so many sandwiched caregivers, I was always afraid of dropping those balls. The average caregiver is a forty-nine-year-old woman who spends twenty hours a week caring for a parent.[2] Add jobs, kids, and siblings who won't or can't help and you've got a whole lot of juggling going on.

Although plenty of siblings collaborate through the caregiving process, conflict, indifference, and childhood wounds that stubbornly resurface divide others. Studies indicate that 45 percent of adults have a rivalrous or strained relationship with their siblings.[3] Those long-smoldering resentments may combust when parents start to decline.

Disagreements about what's best for your mother—remaining at home, moving in with your sister, or going to a nursing home—can lead to all-out battles. One of the most stressful aspects of caring for parents is trying to get on the same page with your brothers and sisters. How do you bring them in when they are just watching (and weighing in) from the sidelines? When is it time to cut them loose? How do you form a team so you are not the go-to person for everything? Can you let go of your need to control things and let others take over, even if they don't do as good a job? The fact that your kid brother always got away with murder should not, but often does, add fuel to the current dilemma about how best to care for your parents.

There may be days you want to bottle your frustrations in a jar and hurl them at your brother or sister. But don't resort to cracking skulls, because two heads are often better than one. With a little patience, perspective, and humor, you can stay focused on what's best for your loved one and find a path forward together.

Alpha Daughters

When it feels like you are the only person you can rely on, it's hard to let go. Mallory fit the profile of an average caregiver, but nothing in her life felt normal. At forty-eight, she was sandwiched between a rock and a hard place. The rock was her eighty-seven-year-old mother, who lived alone and whose health and memory had been declining for years. Despite Mallory's coaxing and pleading, her mother refused to leave her small row home in a suburb outside of New York City, an hour from where Mallory lived. The hard place was Mallory's fifteen-year-old daughter Maya, whose stormy adolescence had turned into a full-blown maelstrom. As a single working mother and only daughter, Mallory was a stretched-thin caregiver on two fronts. She alone shouldered the worry for her daughter, who struggled with learning disabilities. She alone oversaw the day-to-day care of her mother, whose diminishing health was an increasing source of stress.

Mallory had a younger brother, Max, but he lived quite a distance away and was not much help. Proximity is a strong predictor of becoming a caregiver.[4] If you live within a two-hour drive and your sibling lives a plane ride away, chances are you're it. Where was Mallory's brother when she needed him? On the West Coast, three thousand miles away and too busy to find time to pitch in with Mom's care or even pick up the phone to check in.

According to Emily Saltz, founder and CEO of Life Care Advocates, a care management practice serving elderly clients and their families, and past president of the

Aging Life Care Association, sibling conflicts can significantly intensify during an eldercare crisis. Saltz describes the classic primary caregiver as "a daughter who is resentful that her siblings are not helping out. Sometimes the daughter is so in charge and competent that the siblings become passive and let her do all the work." Such was the case with Mallory and Max. Even as a kid, Mallory was given more chores and expected to perform better in school than her artistic, "happy-go-lucky" brother. Growing up, Mallory resented the fact that Max got a free pass on childhood responsibilities. Years later, Max moved to L.A. to pursue an acting career and seemed to leave his family behind. When he did swoop in during a rare visit with his mother, Max failed to ask if there was anything he could do to help. There was plenty. Instead, he would take his mother to dinner and the theater (on Mom's dime). Then he'd return home without any idea of how tough things were. Max's visits always seemed to uplift his mother, who would praise him for taking time out of his busy schedule. Yet Mallory's ongoing efforts to care for her mother barely elicited a thank-you.

Caregivers like Mallory, who feel unappreciated, tend to have less collaborative and more problematic relationships with their siblings.[5] At times Mallory felt invisible. She resented Max, who barely acknowledged that their mother needed help, let alone that Mallory was the one providing it. As her burdens increased, so did Mallory's pent-up frustration. Between managing her mother's care and Maya's schedule, Mallory's life seemed like an endless series of must-dos. Meanwhile Mom appeared to be growing more forgetful by the day. During one visit, Mallory's mother referred to Mallory as Max, which was both irritating and alarming. After an exhausting week of shuttling between homes, Mallory called Max and let him have it. "She's your mother too!" Mallory bellowed. "Now do your fair share and help out!" Mallory laid bare her emotions—the anger, fear, and sadness that had been submerged for too long. Max was surprised, concerned, and contrite. He had thought Mallory had it under control. She'd never expressly asked for help. Max had assumed that his older sister, who lived nearby—and was, after all, the daughter—would be the go-to person when their mother needed care.

Families all too often assign the role of caregiver through a "default" position.[6] They assume the child most likely to be the caregiver is the only daughter, the oldest son, the one close by, the favorite, the most functional, or the least likely to make waves. There are a whole host of reasons one child steps into the caregiving role within families, and most of the time these reasons are unspoken. Simmering conflicts can lead to long-standing feuds when care is proportioned based on assumption rather than open communication. While men are increasingly stepping up as caregivers, historically this role has been assumed by women. And women have not always been great at asking for help.

Since Mallory had to be self-reliant for so long, stepping back and letting go were not her sweet spots. She jokingly said she had OCD—"overcompetence disorder" —but was "in recovery." Max was willing to be more involved in their mother's care, but Mallory needed to apportion tasks and lower her expectations. First, she had to realize her brother's "fair share" did not mean an equal share, but Max could be more involved and lessen Mallory's burden all the same. So, during one visit, Max repaired a leaky faucet, shopped for groceries, and took Mom to the neurologist. Mallory noted that Max had purchased regular produce, not the requested organic variety, but she didn't mention it and praised him anyway. Max, in turn, found ways to thank Mallory through words and deeds. On her forty-ninth birthday, Max surprised Mallory with Broadway tickets to *The Book of Mormon*. Mallory and Maya had a cherished mother/daughter evening together, a much-needed reprieve from the stress of their everyday lives.

Although tensions occasionally flared, Max and Mallory were able to work things out and find common ground. They tried to stay focused and not let past hurts throw them off course. They weaned their mother from her overreliance on Mallory as the go-to person for everything and introduced an in-home caregiver. While Max pitched in more than he once had, the burden of care remained largely on Mallory's shoulders.

When their mother was dying, Mallory called Max to come right away. He did not. Max had the lead in a show and promised he would come as soon as the performance was over—but by the time the curtain had closed, their mother had passed away. Mallory was hurt and angry. She expressed her feelings to Max but chose not to let them fester. Mallory came to accept her brother's limitations, realizing she had no control over how Max chose to cope with the loss of their mother. Max had been distant long before their mother's death and was even more so now. While Mallory no longer needed help from her brother, she yearned for more connection.

So she found it elsewhere and joined a caregiver support group, where she shared her experience and developed strong bonds. Mallory and fellow group members discussed their struggles over end of life care, money, and family allocation of responsibility. Mallory was gratified to find she could help others who felt isolated, and whose siblings were not always willing or able to share the care-giving role.

The Impaired Sibling

Mallory had always been labeled the responsible one in her family and Max the free spirit—limited perhaps, but able to function on his own. What about siblings who suffer from disabilities that prevent them from managing their own lives effectively, never mind anyone else's? Some people are faced with a double whammy: caring for a parent in decline and negotiating the emotional and financial needs of an impaired sibling.

Cara knew this dual challenge all too well. Her brother Fred had a tumultuous childhood and adolescence, barely making it through high school. In his forties, he suffered from an intractable case of shingles that left him in chronic pain. In Cara's opinion, Fred also suffered from arrested development. As an adult, Fred was still dependent on their mother for support. When Cara's mother developed Alzheimer's disease, that dependency took a worrisome turn. Fred began treating his mother like a "cash cow." Cara recalled her despair over the fact that her mother could no longer make rational decisions, particularly involving finances. She wanted to help her son and that help translated into money. "My mom was bleeding money to Fred before I took over," Cara lamented.

Emily Saltz has worked with many adult siblings whose caregiving conflicts are focused on money issues. "Money symbolizes control," explains Saltz. "When siblings struggle over financial issues, they often stop focusing on what is best for their parents." This can be particularly challenging when there is a disabled sibling. Elder law attorneys can offer solutions through estate planning, special needs trusts, and financial management. Cara solved the problem by obtaining power of attorney, giving her the authority to make financial decisions on her mother's behalf. Fred was initially hurt and resistant to the idea. Cara made sure Fred received a monthly stipend but no longer had access to Mom's finances. "I made all the decisions because my brother was not capable of doing so. It actually made things easier," explained Cara.

In some cases, the impaired sibling insists on playing a role in a parent's care and that's when things can get thorny. Roger's older sister Brett always seemed to upset the apple cart. Brett's depression and unpredictable mood swings would send their mother, recently diagnosed with Parkinson's disease, into a tailspin. Research studies indicate that an adult child's emotional difficulties can increase the risk of psychological distress on a mother, further complicating caregiving relationships.[7] Roger's mother was considering a move to assisted living when Brett went ballistic over losing her childhood home. Brett also expressed concern about her inheritance. "This is not about you!" Roger insisted. "Mom is not safe in that big old house and all you care about is yourself." Brett offered to take care of their mother but that approach backfired. The more time Brett spent with her mother, the more Mom worried about her daughter. Roger felt he needed to take care of both his mother and sister, but his efforts were met by resistance on both fronts.

Sometimes siblings like Roger and Brett are so polarized they are not able to move forward with any type of plan. When that happens, it may be time to bring in eldercare mediators, professionals who help families work through disputes and achieve consensus in eldercare decisions. Roger hired a mediator who met with everyone individually at first, including Roger's mother. By the time a family meeting took place, there was a unifying theme. Roger and Brett's mother needed daily care, and neither sibling could provide that. Brett eventually gave up her objections to selling the house, and her mother was willing to move to a more suitable community. Roger and Brett had finally become unstuck, but they needed an outside facilitator to make that happen.

According to Arline Kardasis and Crystal Thorpe, co-founders of Elder Decisions, a nationally recognized mediation and consulting firm specializing in adult family conflict resolution, disagreements can quickly escalate, particularly in issues related to inheritance. "We facilitate a conversation," explain Kardasis and Thorpe. "We don't take sides or give advice." Mediators get everyone's perspective, including the senior's, and help families consider different options and work toward shared goals. "It's important to respect the elder's wishes while building consensus within the family." In some cases, that means casting a wide net and including spouses and grandchildren. When hiring mediators, do your homework and ask for a referral from a trusted source such as an elder law attorney. Prices vary widely across the country, between $100 and $500 an hour, but the service can save families costly and fractious litigation.

As Roger and Brett learned, imbalances in emotional, psychological, and financial resources can complicate sibling caregiver relationships. In some families these disparities may lead to greater clarity over who does what. One sibling must assume the role of caregiver because the other still needs to be cared for. Assessing a sibling's strengths and limitations is not straightforward. Siblings are insecure. They have blind spots and think they don't need help—or they ask for support, then push it away. They feel threatened when other family members invade their caregiving turf. How do you get your brother to accept help and not make himself and everyone around him miserable? It's not so easy, especially if he lives far away and you're also negotiating your father's care from a distance.

The Help Seeker/Help Rejecter

Years ago families more or less stayed in one place. Children grew up, planted roots in their hometown, and brothers and sisters (mostly sisters) would share the care of their elders when the time came. Nowadays, far-flung siblings negotiate the messy terrain of caring for their aging parents from afar. Getting on the same page can be more challenging when you are not in the same place— physically or emotionally. Guilt and guesswork can muddy the waters; perhaps one sibling feels guilty for not being around and second-guesses the other sibling who is. This can lead to the so-called Seagull Syndrome, wherein the long-distance sibling swoops in and craps all over the caregiving sibling's plan, increasing the emotional divide. In some cases, the caregiving sibling becomes entrenched and stubbornly refuses to accept help despite repeated offers. That's when some family members may take matters into their own hands.

Rick constantly complained to his brother and sister-in-law about their lack of involvement with his father's care. Rick lived in Maryland and cared for his father at home while his brother and family lived in Oregon. The bicoastal distance exacerbated an already tense standoff. Rick's brother felt that money paid to in-home caregivers would be better spent on assisted living. Rick insisted his dad would never agree to a move and his brother just needed to chip in more time and money. After a year of squabbling, Rick's brother and his wife had had enough. They flew to Maryland, presented Dad with an option of assisted living, and took him back to Oregon, overriding Rick's objections. To Rick's surprise, his father adjusted readily to the new surroundings—within a few weeks, he even had a girlfriend at the assisted living community.

Rick had been a stuck caregiver. He resented his brother and sister-in-law for not doing enough, but refused to consider their offer to help. Rick's brother felt increasingly guilty and frustrated. Eventually he and his wife wrestled control away from Rick, who was not ready to relinquish the caregiver role. Dealing with a help-seeking/help-rejecting sibling caregiver can feel like damned if you do, damned if you don't. In some cases, siblings like Rick's brother may choose to act, pushing through resistance and moving full steam ahead. Other families may choose to do nothing and let the help-rejecting caregiver stew in his or her own juices. Both approaches are problematic. Ideally, addressing the sibling's help-seeking and help-rejecting pattern honestly, empathically, and tactfully works best. Show appreciation for all that your sibling does, reiterate that you want what's right for your parent, and communicate that your offer to help is being rebuffed. Avoid generic overtures such as "Let me know if there is anything I can do" and agree on specific tasks that will ease your sibling's burden.

The Lonely Onlys

In her work with caregivers over the past twenty-five years, Emily Saltz, who has seen a lot of siblings "swirl in past hurts," says the real task is refocusing energy on what's best for the parent. "The worst thing for your parent is to know you are fighting about them." How about caregivers who have no siblings at all? "There's good news and bad news," says Saltz. "The bad news is that it's all on you. The good news is that you have no one to negotiate with or block your plan." The percentage of couples with just one child has doubled over the past twenty years, according to the Pew Research Center.[8] There are many stereotypes associated with only children—narcissism, increased intelligence, and self-absorption, to name a few.

There seems to be no agreement about the advantages and disadvantages of being an only child, but when it comes to caring for aging parents, you are on your own. "It can be quite isolating and lonely at times," says James, a fifty-seven-year-old Chinese American whose parents emigrated from China as young adults. As a professor of molecular biology at a prestigious university, James had a respected position that provided him with a sense of accomplishment and control. "But when it came to helping out my parents, I felt like a child."

Filial piety has always been a core value of the Chinese culture, explained James. It's a Confucian belief that adult children are obligated to care for their parents, both emotionally and materially. Now in China, following an only-child policy that was recently relaxed, it is also the law. A report examining the psychological well-being of Chinese Americans caring for their aging parents links an increase in anxiety and depression with the pressures of filial piety.[9] This strong cultural mandate is then layered on top of the ordinary stress of caregiving.

James acknowledged feeling stressed by the demands of caregiving with no siblings to chip in or play interference. "I can stand in front of a room of experts and expound on the intricacies of molecular genetics," says James. "But I can't get my parents to accept any help in their home besides me. I had no one to turn to and help me deal with my parents' demands." Eventually James found support from a senior care expert. "She was better than a sibling in some ways," explains James. "She was objective, knowledgeable, and was always in my corner." James discovered that being an only child did not have to mean being alone. Ultimately he joined a support group and developed a sibship of sorts with his fellow caregivers. "Our experiences may have been different but our struggles were similar. I felt sad and afraid a lot of the time. Once I reached out for help, I was less alone. But I first had to come to terms with my parents' fallibility—and my own."

Family Harmony Is a Glorified Ideal

In her book *They're Your Parents, Too! How Siblings Can Survive Their Parents' Aging without Driving Each Other Crazy*, Francine Russo describes the Norman Rockwell ideal, "the flawless fantasy family that exists only in the imagination, the standard against which so many adults measure the less-than-perfect family in which they grew up."[10] This tendency toward idealization, according to Russo, can lead us to magical thinking. We imagine our siblings will rally and shed their baggage as we join forces to care for our parents. Yet unresolved conflicts can get dragged into the present and past wounds exposed. If we have not worked through our differences, we must put them aside as much as possible. We must also learn to ask for help and be realistic about our siblings' limitations. If your brother doesn't like to get involved, don't expect him to take charge after your mother has a stroke. Don't look to your anxious sister to model self-composure after your father's health declines. Keep your expectations in check. Like James and Mallory, seek supports elsewhere when your own brothers and sisters fall short.

Communication Matters

When you're overwhelmed and overburdened, it's easy to feel that your siblings are standing on the sideline taking potshots. Those on the front lines of caregiving may not say it, but they need support, encouragement, and all hands on deck. Feeling criticized doesn't help. This can lead to the "I shouldn't have to ask" phenomenon. Yes, you should. And you should speak up when you feel ignored, dismissed, and abandoned. Don't let it simmer until you burst.

Communication can be further complicated when there are three or more of you. Someone always seems to get left out. Growing up, my brother, sister, and I used to play a game that seems pretty mean in retrospect. When the three of us were together, one would start the game by saying, "Funny, but there are only two people in this room. The other one must be a rock." The designated "rock" would then be totally ignored while the other two siblings played happily together. With adult children, the rock can transform into a giant iceberg, sinking the plans of the more collaborative siblings. While not all siblings can participate equally, it is important to establish a plan of communication that everyone agrees on. Technology can help. Some families use email, Skype, or regularly scheduled conference calls. A website called Lotsa Helping Hands (www.lotsahelpinghands.com) provides an online secure community for caregivers to coordinate and organize information such as appointments, medications, finances, and day-to-day tasks. Online tools are especially useful when siblings are scattered across the country or the globe.

Don't Be an Air Traffic Controller

Effective communication strategies can shift the burden of responsibility from the alpha daughter (or son) to other family members, including the senior. In some families, one child serves as the parental interpreter and translates Mom's or Dad's wishes and frustrations to the other siblings. When you see yourself as air traffic control, taking on the role of communicator-in-chief, you may ultimately make things worse. Rather than ensuring a smooth landing, you are likely to increase the odds of a collision. If your mother complains your sister is never around, let Mom tell your sister that herself. If your father resents your brother's intrusiveness, don't play referee. Caregiving may fan the flames of long-standing conflicts between parents and their adult children. Focus on what can be done to help your parents in the present rather than attempt to heal old wounds from the past. If you sidestep getting triangulated in family disputes, you may avoid some of the grief, guilt, and guesswork of trying to solve a problem you can't fix.

The Fight to Be Right

One of the biggest areas of conflict between siblings is the different perception of parents' needs and how best to approach care. Exchanges like these happen in many families:

> "Our father's getting really forgetful. I'm worried that he can't be left alone anymore."
>
> "Dad's fine. For eighty-five, I think he's doing okay."
>
> "It's not safe for Mom to live at home anymore. We need to think about nursing homes."

"Over my dead body! We promised our mother we would take care of her at home."

Guilt may also be a driver in decision making, especially for the sibling who isn't around as much and feels the need to step in. The right kind of professional guidance may help minimize conflict and provide you and your family with some realistic solutions. Aging life care professionals can conduct on-site assessments of a senior's ability to manage safely at home and can recommend resources and home modifications. When hiring an aging life care professional, discuss how information will be shared between you and your siblings. Will you be given a written report or a verbal summary? Will you and your siblings review recommendations before you discuss them with your parent? These professionals must form a trusting bond with elders to develop a mutually agreeable plan of care. They can also help you and your siblings stop struggling over who is right and instead focus on what works best.

Let It Go

As any ten-year-old fan of *Frozen* can tell you, sometimes you just gotta "let it go." When it comes to sibling resentments, we hold on to things that happened a lifetime ago. Meanwhile, our parents may not make it any easier.

Your mother stokes resentment when she moans about your brother to you but not to him. Your dad relies on your all-suffering sister, who complains bitterly but can never say no. And Mom won't ask your brother who lives nearby to take her to the doctor because she says he's too busy. As if you're not. Years ago at a seminar I was giving about siblings and caregiving a young woman spoke to me about her brother. She had tried everything imaginable to get him to participate in her mother's care. As a lawyer, she had even threatened him with legal action. Despite numerous efforts, nothing she said or did had any impact. Her brother was either completely unwilling or unable to be a caregiver. It was a painful reality this woman had to acknowledge before she could move forward with a plan. "Let it go," I said. "Your brother is not going to help. You need to find other sources of support and accept his limitations." She let go of her quest for fairness and instead focused on what was attainable. Understanding the root cause of the imbalance may help. In this woman's case, her brother had been the "black sheep," disappointing their parents for dropping out of college and getting in scuffles with the law. While that doesn't excuse him from responsibility, it put things in perspective. "He received more anger from my folks, whereas I got more praise," the woman noted. "He may have had less available to give."

Life-Long Bond

Recently my family and a host of friends celebrated my sister's sixtieth birthday. My brother put together a slide show that captured hilarious and poignant slices of my sister's life throughout the decades. Birthday parties, vacations, graduations, and family gatherings—sixty years of life melded into a beautiful montage. Many people in the photos, like my father, are not with us anymore. Others, such as aunts, cousins, and friends, continue to make up the closely woven tapestry of our family life. As birthdays continue to come and go, many others who were present will be gone. That unspoken reality has brought my brother, sister, and me closer together, knowing that it is up to us to be the torchbearers. We will pass on our parents' legacies and life lessons to our children. We share a collective memory that is unique to us, a memory that becomes more precious even as it grows dimmer.

In his thought-provoking book *Sibling Relationships across the Life Span*, psychologist Victor Cicirelli, PhD, reveals a powerful truth: the most enduring relationships in our life are with our brothers and sisters. It is not unusual, according to Cicirelli, to know our siblings twice as long as our parents.[11] This knowledge may cement sibling bonds and help us get past the fissures that may accumulate as we grow into adulthood. Our shared memories, both the good and the bad, have the power to transcend our differences. I am immensely grateful that my brother, sister, and I were able to support each other during the course of my father's dementia. There were many tough times—late-night vigils in the emergency room and the slow, steady progression of a debilitating disease that gradually took my father's life. But there were also shared joys, laughter, sing-alongs with Dad in the nursing home, and the remarkable gift of being truly present with one another. My siblings and I traveled this life-changing road together, and we've continued to uphold and cherish our father's memory since he's been gone. That is the gift of having siblings in your life. There may be quarrels and conflicts, but there are also healthy and healing ways to work out your differences and help your parents age with dignity, compassion, and love.

FIVE

What Does Care Cost, and Who Pays?

> Money's only something you need in case you
> don't die tomorrow.
> —CARL FOX (MARTIN SHEEN) IN *WALL STREET*

Many of us have read the titillating and tragic story of
Sumner Redstone, the former head of Viacom, and the li-
tigious financial power struggle that embroiled his family.
It involved a lot of money, a dementing and pugnacious
media mogul, a conniving former lover, and a daughter
trying to wrest control of the family fortune from a sor-
did mess.[1] Most of us won't need to worry about a multi-
billion-dollar empire, and our family struggles may appear mundane by comparison. But disagreements over
money can and often do prevent families from making

the right choices about care. Unresolved financial conflicts may live on long after a parent is gone. The good news is that you and your family can come up with a game plan before a crisis erupts. Remember the Scout's mantra: Be prepared! Understanding the confounding landscape of what is or is not covered by insurance can help families approach caregiving with forethought and compassion —no matter what the cost. As crude as it may seem, having financial resources—or not—may determine your available options and the type of long-term care you ultimately receive.

A big shocker for many is that Medicare, the primary insurer for 55 million older adults and people with disabilities, does not typically pay for long-term care services. That includes nursing homes, which are covered by Medicaid, but only for those who are eligible. The tough reality is that many families aren't rich enough to afford the staggering cost of long-term care but don't qualify for Medicaid either. That was the case with my father, who spent six years in two different nursing homes. If you are among the "in-betweeners," you'll need to be resourceful and possibly dig deep into your pockets because care is expensive. There's a lot to learn and what you don't know *can* hurt you.

If you are caring for a parent outside the United States,

you will need to do some research into that country's system of long-term care. In the United Kingdom, for example, many people assume the National Health System will pay for long-term care, but many families end up funding care themselves or relying on cash-strapped localities. In Canada, coverage for long-term care varies widely by provinces and territories. Japan, which has one of the fastest-growing populations of older adults in the world, introduced a mandatory long-term care insurance system in 2000 to lessen the burden on family caregivers. While the family, most often a daughter or daughter-in-law, still provides the majority of care, home- and community-based services can offer much-needed assistance and respite.

What, Me Worry?

Any boomer worth his or her weight in salt can recall the motto of *Mad* magazine's famed mascot, Alfred E. Neumann. Now that boomers are turning sixty-five at a rate of ten thousand people a day, it may be time to worry, at least about what comes next.[2] Seventy percent of Americans over age sixty-five will need some form of long-term care support during their lifetime.[3] Although most won't end up in nursing homes like my dad, many may need in-home care at some point. My mother cared for my father at home for six years—until she couldn't anymore. She was among the 80 percent of family caregivers who provide the vast majority of unpaid care in this country, valued at $470 billion annually.[4]

According to the annual Genworth cost of care survey, people consistently underestimate the cost of long-term care.[5] Boomers in typical "What, me worry?" fashion are also more optimistic about their own future health than they should be. Jeff Goldsmith, a healthcare futurist and author of *The Long Baby Boom: An Optimistic Vision for a Graying Generation*, claims this optimism is unfounded.[6] There is a mismatch between boomers' predictions of their health in retirement and the reality. In a recent poll, only 13 percent of those surveyed predicted their health would worsen in retirement, compared with 39 percent who said their health actually deteriorated after they retired.[7] Many of us may be on the golf course or doing downward-facing dog poses well into our eighties, but when it comes to aging, one should hope for the best and plan for the worst.

Can We Talk?

"Can we talk?" the inimitable Joan Rivers asked before lacerating her subject matter with acerbic humor. While a little levity might be helpful, it's best to be calm and compassionate when approaching delicate conversations about money. Yes, you should talk, but it's one of those uncomfortable topics that adult children and their parents often avoid—to everyone's detriment. Viewing money as a private matter is ingrained in our culture, particularly for the generation that came of age during World War II. But it is precisely these candid conversations that enable family caregivers to chart a pragmatic course based on realistic options. It's best to bring up money as part of a series of conversations about planning ahead—for better *and* for worse. Even if your father is hale and hearty, he's likely to need help one day. And that help costs money.

Recently my husband and I redid our wills. Our kids are all in their twenties so the focus is less on them and more on us. According to Harry Margolis, a seasoned elder law attorney and managing partner of Margolis & Bloom in Boston, people tend to think about their wills when their children are small, then not again until they're considering retirement. Having parents who had to slog through the quagmire of long-term care can be another motivator. I know what care costs and what decisions need to be made. Should something happen to us, my husband and I don't want our kids sorting it out on their own. So we sat our three children down and had the "What if?" conversation. We discussed scary topics like nursing homes

(I would rather go to a nice one than have them care for me). We told them when to pull the plug, we asked them not to fight over the beach house, and we talked openly about money (at least, what's left after all their college tuitions). We designated our oldest son as our durable power of attorney, giving him authority to make financial and health-related decisions should we both become incapacitated. These are not fun topics to discuss. The conversation may evolve as our needs change, but we kick-started the dialogue by bringing it up early.

When families avoid this topic entirely, decisions tend to be made based on urgency. Those decisions typically involve personal finances. Don't be surprised if an inquiry into your mother's bank account is met with resistance. David Solie, author of *How to Say It to Seniors*, cites fear of loss of control as a primary driver for older adults. Adult children tend to exacerbate this fear by approaching delicate conversations with demands and admonitions ("You have to . . .," "You can't . . .," "If you don't . . ."). Even broaching the topic of personal finances can feel infantilizing for seniors, especially when it's tied to needing care one day. Solie suggests positioning yourself as a supportive helper rather than an enforcer and phrasing your concern in a way that doesn't take control away from your parent.[8] Try sharing information you learned about long-term care facts and figures: "I just read an interesting article about the rising cost of care and it got me thinking . . ." Or shift the focus away from your parents by mentioning your friend's sticker shock over home care costs. Perhaps you updated your own estate planning and can use that as a springboard for conversation. Before you dive into the money talk, do your homework. Learn the difference between Medicare and Medicaid. Find out if your parents have long-term care insurance or if they were veterans. If so, they may be eligible for veterans benefits, which could save a boatload of money. Once you know the basics, you'll know what to ask and where to go for answers.

Medicare and Medicaid: Get Them Straight

Frank was ill prepared when his mother died suddenly and left him the sole caregiver of his eighty-six-year-old father with Alzheimer's disease. When Frank began to explore nursing homes, he was startled by the price tag: $85,000 a year! "I had mistakenly thought Medicare would pay for a nursing home. Apparently Medicare only pays for short-term care and my father didn't qualify for that. When I finally got my parents' finances straight, it was bleak. There was little savings and no long-term care insurance. They were 'over income' for Medicaid but didn't have money to pay for a nursing home either. I wish we had started the process of planning much sooner." Frank hired an elder law attorney. Only then was he able to sort out the finances, get his father on a Medicaid "spend-down" and use the existing private pay funds for care right away.

Frank is not alone in his uncertainty. Medicare and Medicaid are often confused, and the similarity of their names doesn't help. Both are governmental programs created by Lyndon Johnson as part of his "Great Society" vision in 1965. Recently celebrating fiftieth anniversaries, Medicaid and Medicare were designed to improve the health, well-being, and economic security of all Americans. Boy, have these programs grown! Medicaid has swelled from a mere 4 million in 1966 to over 74 million recipients today.[9] In 1966, Medicare covered a little over 19 million Americans compared to 56 million today.[10] The most dramatic growth has been recently, as the generation that once advised, "Never trust anyone over thirty" signs up for Medicare in record numbers.

Despite the large reach of both these programs, when it comes to paying for long-term care, there is a lot of confusion. Medicare is a federally funded insurance program for people age sixty-five and older, regardless of income. It was expanded in 1972 to include people with disabilities.[11] Medicare has four parts: hospital costs, skilled nursing, home health, and hospice (Part A); outpatient services and medical supplies (Part B); Medicare Advantage Plans offered by private insurers (Part C); and prescription drug coverage (Part D), which was added in 2003.

One of the best resources to learn more about Medicare coverage and eligibility is the Medicare.gov website (www.medicare.gov). Another, more user-friendly site is www.medicareinteractive.org. You can also speak to a SHIP (state health insurance program) counselor at no charge. Funded by the U.S. Department of Health and Human Services, SHIP counselors (also known as SHINE in some states) are mostly volunteers who can walk you through the ABCs of Medicare. They can explain what Medicare does and does not cover, when to buy supplemental insurance such as Medigap, and what Medicare plan may be best for you (original or Medicare Advantage). But plan ahead. If you call around the Medicare open enrollment period, October 15–December 7, you may have a long wait.

Medicaid is funded jointly by states and the federal government, which means that rules vary depending on where you live. Even the term *Medicaid* has its own brand name in many states. It's called Husky Health in Connecticut, BadgerCare in Wisconsin, and the pastoral Green Mountain Care in Vermont. Medicaid is the largest funding source for long-term care in nursing homes. Unlike Medicare, which covers everyone regardless of income, Medicaid is for people with low incomes, who typically have no more than $2,000 in "countable" assets. This is where things get tricky. There are some assets that count and others that don't. There are ways to transfer certain assets years ahead of time. That means your father has to trust you with his money or property a full five years before he may need a nursing home.

You can also spend down assets toward "medically necessary" expenses that can qualify you for Medicaid. That could include hospital bills or medications not otherwise covered by insurance. It could also mean a prepaid funeral plan with some specific guidelines—sort of a tough topic to bring up at a family get-together. Harry Margolis, founder of Elder Law Answers (elderlawanswers.com), urges families to plan in advance as much as possible. If you haven't sorted out finances ahead of time, however, don't despair, Margolis says. "Once the event happens there is still a lot an elder law attorney can do to help you sort out Medicaid eligibility and the cost of long-term care."

If your parents are sixty-five years or older and are U.S. citizens, they probably have Medicare. If they end up qualifying for rehabilitation after a hospital stay,

Medicare will pay for up to one hundred days of skilled care in a skilled nursing facility (also known as a SNF— pronounced *snif*). These rehab stays often take place in actual nursing homes, which are geared for people who need a slower pace, like my father. But don't get confused. If your father no longer has a need for daily skilled help— time's up, whether he's been there for a hundred days or not. To be eligible for rehab under Medicare, patients must have a need for skilled care—nursing, physical therapy, speech therapy, or occupational therapy. They must demonstrate the capacity for improvement or the likelihood that skilled care will prevent further deterioration. If these conditions aren't met, Medicare coverage may end.

Another maddening loophole under Medicare that catches families off guard is the phenomenon of "observation status": patients who spend time in the hospital but are not technically admitted. Why does that matter? Medicare requires a three-day inpatient hospitalization in order to qualify for care in a skilled nursing facility after discharge. Observation status is considered outpatient (Part B), so if your family member needs post-hospital nursing coverage, you'll be digging deep into your pockets because Medicare won't pay. If you or your loved ones land in the hospital under observation, time to be a squeaky wheel. You will need to convince the healthcare team that the hospital stay is medically necessary, and you may want to recruit your primary care physician to help make the case. You can also contact the Center for Medicare Advocacy (www. medicareadvocacy.org) for guidelines on what action to take if this happens to you.

Rehab to Nursing Home

Considering a transition from rehab to nursing home care can be a tough decision for families, as it was for mine. Several years into my father's dementia, he became incontinent. My mother had previously been able to handle most aspects of Dad's care on her own. But when my father could no longer bathe or go to the bathroom by himself, it was a game changer. With Mom's added physical challenge, we began to worry about her too. To make matters worse, my father got frequent urinary tract infections (UTIs). UTIs can cause confusion (in fact, they are sometimes mistaken as early signs of Alzheimer's and other forms of dementia) and can lead to life-threatening infections. My father couldn't tell us when he had a UTI, but we learned the telltale signs. He withdrew, became noncommunicative and, perhaps most uncharacteristic of all, he lost his appetite.

During one bout with a UTI, my father ended up in the

hospital. Once stabilized, he was transferred to a rehab unit within an area nursing home where he received physical therapy to regain his strength. My father was cooperative with the physical therapists, many of them engaging young women whom he greeted with his characteristic charm. The care was good and my father improved. While short-term rehabilitation and long-term nursing care are often housed under one roof, the quality of care may not be the same. That was the case with this facility. In the nursing home unit, listless residents in wheelchairs were lined up in the activity room and plunked in front of a television airing cartoons all day. The staff appeared distracted and apathetic. After my father had made sufficient progress and was no longer eligible for rehab, we had to make a decision: take him home or transfer him to the long-term care unit? While there was a bed available, I didn't have a good feeling about the place. Like most people with advanced dementia, my father was not capable of clearly expressing his opinion. But I gave it a shot anyway. "Dad," I said, "on a scale of one to ten, how would you rate this place? Let's say ten is the Ritz Carlton and one is a crappy motel." My father appeared to be pondering the question for a while. Then he responded, "Three." "Why only three?" I asked. My father couldn't articulate what was wrong, but he knew the difference between good and bad care. "This is no way to run a railroad," he explained.

We had our answer. We took him home.

Home Sweet Home Care

Up until this time, caring for my father was a family affair. Once in a while, a neighbor or friend came by to keep an eye on Dad, but otherwise my mother did it all, with occasional help from me and my siblings. My brother, sister, and I had suggested home care as a way to give my mom a much-needed break. But my mother, like many family caregivers, didn't want to spend the money. Home care, whether provided by a paid caregiver or a family member, is foundational to human existence. It's food in the fridge and clean clothes to wear, a helping hand to guide you out of the chair without falling. Families do so much of this. But they can't do it all. Those who have received this type of assistance from a compassionate and skilled caregiver know its worth. But many families simply can't afford it.

Nonmedical home care, the type of care my father needed, is typically not covered by Medicare, and the median cost is around $20 an hour (in some states it is considerably more). There is no federal oversight of nonmedical home care. Some states have licensure requirements; others don't. There are different types of in-home caregivers you can hire: homemakers, also known as companion caregivers, who help with laundry, meal prep, socialization, and errands; and home health aides and CNAs (certified nursing assistants), who are trained to provide hands-on personal care such as bathing, dressing, and toileting. Most people pay privately for nonmedical home care and the cost can quickly add up. In some cases, nonmedical home care is covered by Medicaid under the Medicaid waiver program. This allows state Medicaid programs to divert funds that might otherwise be spent on nursing homes (a costlier option). The Area Agencies on Aging can give you information about state-specific programs that are designed to help frail elders live in the community rather than a nursing home. Although families may still need to provide some level of care, Medicaid waiver programs can help those who are eligible to remain at home. Given the current firestorm around healthcare funding in the United States, support for these programs, which so many people rely on, is more precarious than ever.

Luz Jiménez, a fifty-two-year-old Colombian immigrant struggling to care for her mother on a housekeeper's salary, was no stranger to hardship. In 1995, at the age of thirty-two, Luz came to the United States to escape the Medellín drug cartel. Her husband was not so lucky. According to Luz, he was murdered "by mistake," a random killing in a country ravaged by violence. Once Luz became a U.S. citizen, she focused on her next priority—getting her mother out of Colombia. A family immigration petition was eventually granted and Luz was thrilled to have her mother close by again. "She took care of me when I was younger. I want to do the same. I say to God, please give me time with my mother. Don't take her away." But something had changed, and Luz's mother was not the same. She repeated herself endlessly, became easily agitated, and could no longer make her signature tamales. Luz was bereft when a doctor diagnosed her mother with Alzheimer's disease. What was Luz to do? She worked full-time for a commercial cleaning company. She could barely make ends meet as it was. While Luz was eventually able to get her mother on Medicaid, Luz refused to consider a nursing home. "It is how I was raised," said Luz. "We take care of our own."

Luz is among the many family caregivers who dip into their own pockets to pay for care. She paid for medicine, medical co-pays, and other necessities like adult diapers. Studies show that family caregivers spend close to $7,000 annually on out-of-pocket caregiving costs not covered by insurance.[12] For Luz, that was a big chunk of her take-home pay. Luz reached out to her local Area Agency on

Aging hoping her mother could get some type of support. Luz's mother, whose dementia made her eligible for nursing home care, qualified for a home-based program called PACE (program for all-inclusive care for the elderly), which is available in some states. PACE is designed to help people with Medicare and Medicaid receive care in the community instead of a nursing home or other institutional setting. For Luz, it was a life saver. Her mother had access to services such as case management (a social worker who coordinated services and supported Luz), Meals on Wheels and, most important—home care. Nonmedical home care essentially kept Luz's mother out of a nursing home and allowed her to stay at home with Luz. That's the type of day-to-day care that is so vital. But since it's considered custodial (not skilled), it is not covered by Medicare. Does Medicare ever cover nonmedical home care like a home health aide? Sometimes it does, but usually not for long.

Home Health Care: Here Today, Gone Tomorrow

Six months after my father died, my mother fell and broke her femur. She was in the hospital less than three days before being transferred to a rehabilitation facility. After several weeks of rehab, my mother returned home alone. She was in a wheelchair, maneuvering around her house for seven long months. Fortunately, my mother lived in a senior-safe home within a retirement community. Unfortunately, none of her children lived nearby. Knowing that my still-grieving mother had to manage on her own was one of those guilt-inducing experiences we caregivers often face. So my brother, sister, and I descended on my mother's home to try to come up with a plan. We rearranged the furniture so Mom could more easily move about her one-story home in a wheelchair. We organized the fridge so she could have easy access to food—placed wheelchair height on the lower shelf. Since my mom was homebound and had a skilled need (physical therapy), she qualified for home health care through her Medicare benefit. Home health care (also known as Medicare-certified home care) must be ordered by a physician and is defined in this context as care requiring the services of a licensed medical professional such as a nurse, physical therapist, or occupational therapist. Since my mother was stuck in a wheelchair, she could also have a home health aide come twice a day in addition to the physical therapist—all paid for by Medicare. But once my mother could walk a certain distance, essentially hobbling from the bedroom to the bathroom, she was no longer eligible for Medicare-paid home health care. She continued with physical therapy on an outpatient basis but still couldn't drive. What about the aide who helped Mom dress and bathe every day? Mom had reached the point in her recovery when that type of care was no longer covered by Medicare either. What can you do when that happens? You can pay out of pocket or just manage on your own.

Fortunately, my mother could afford a caregiver to help with errands and driving after her Medicare-funded aide was gone. I located a reputable home care agency in the area, but my mother decided to hire a caregiver on her own. Several friends in her retirement community recommended Angela, a Brazilian woman with a strong back and a big heart. Angela had an uncanny knack of knowing when to push and when to back off. She pushed my mother to use her cane more often (something the doctor recommended but that made my mother feel unsteady), and she backed off when my mom needed a break. My mother paid Angela $15 an hour, a greater sum than Angela would have made as a caregiver working for an agency. This arrangement worked well for both Angela and my mother. But hiring a caregiver privately is not right for everyone. Home care agencies don't leave you in the lurch if your caregiver doesn't show up. When deciding whether to hire privately or through a home care agency, it's best to eliminate some of the guesswork and learn the pros and cons of both options ahead of time.

How to Hire a Caregiver

Over the years, I have run a home care agency and I have been a family caregiver. I know what agencies offer and the type of care families need. As an eldercare professional and a family caregiver, I've learned what matters most. Simply put, the best way to receive good care is to hire a really good caregiver. That's what home care agencies are supposed to do. If you hire through an agency you are paying someone to assume the responsibilities of being an employer. You are paying an agency to properly hire, screen, train, supervise, and schedule caregivers. Most agencies will pick a caregiver based on the specified needs of your family member. When the match doesn't work, the agency will have to try again.

Some families prefer to find a paid caregiver on their own. If you hire privately you become the employer. First ask yourself: Can I take this on? It will cost less but it may be more work. Someone needs to be responsible for hiring and vetting the caregiver (including proper background checks). Who's going to make sure your mother's getting the care she needs? When the caregiver needs a day off or doesn't show up at all, who's going to arrange backup care? What happens if the caregiver doesn't click with Mom? You may discover that finding the right caregiver—one your mother doesn't immediately fire—may be no small feat.

Once you decide you want to hire a private caregiver, where do you start? Websites like Care.com offer a platform for families to hire caregivers and tips on how to find the right one. Then there is the issue of paying the caregiver fairly and legally. Most people aren't aware of the complex labor laws and obligations involved with paying domestic workers. Tom Breedlove, director of Homepay, a payroll compliance company within Care .com, says it's important to learn the dos and don'ts of becoming a household employer. "There are a number of financial obligations such as FICA (Social Security and Medicare), withholding and matching, workers' compensation insurance, paid sick leave, and disability as well as tax breaks and benefits—all of which are really important to understand and address correctly at the time of hire," he says. "To make things more confusing, rules vary by state. It may seem overwhelming at first. That's why I recommend hiring a company that specializes in household employment compliance so you can focus on what's most important—being there for your loved one."

Eventually my mother got a device to help her put her socks and shoes on and she no longer needed help from

Angela. After many months, my independent mother was back on her feet again, yet the whole incident was a cautionary tale. She was prone to falls, and falls are the leading cause of injury and death among seniors. So with some encouragement from her kids, my mother joined a weekly Tai Chi and osteoporosis class with the goal of improving her balance and then some. While hoping for the best but planning for the worst, it was important to know that Mom could pay for care if she needed it again. Twenty hours of home care a week at an average cost of $25/hour (based on agency rates in the area) would add up to over $25,000 a year—out of pocket. Fortunately, my mother had purchased a long-term care insurance policy years ago. It was time to find out what it covered and what it didn't—just in case she needed to use it one day.

Who Needs It? Long-Term Care Insurance

Back in the mid-1990s when my parents bought policies, long-term care insurance (LTCI) was steadily on the rise. People like my still relatively healthy parents were willing to fork out some cash to protect themselves against the vagaries of aging. That decision paid off for my dad. Several years later he was diagnosed with dementia. Had he waited, he probably would have been disqualified based on a preexisting (and rather costly) condition.

Many years after the early adapters, like my parents, bought long-term care insurance, they grew old and needed care. Expensive care that was designed to be covered by the very policies they purchased back in the day. Some companies raised their premiums. Others, like the holder of the policy my mother bought, sold to larger companies that changed the rules. And some left the business altogether. Today the American Association for Long-Term Care Insurance shows a dramatic slide in individual market sales of long-term insurance relative to fifteen years ago. Many people don't like the "Use it or lose it" aspect of paying into policies they may never need. That concern has given rise to new models of long-term care insurance, which are hybrid products that combine long-term care funding with permanent life insurance or annuities. If you're in the financial sandwich (too rich for Medicaid but too poor to afford the cost of care), long-term care insurance might be right for you. You'll need to shop around and look into annual premiums, which will vary depending on your age, health status, and type of plan you choose. While you may never need the policy, if you do, you'll be really glad you have it.

Long-term care insurance is essentially a pot of money that you use when you need it, according to the policy's guidelines. There are several options to consider. One of the most important is inflation protection, which allows your benefits to keep pace with the escalating cost of care over many years. Pay attention to maximum daily benefits that limit the amount covered based on your specific policy and the type of care needed. There's also something called an elimination period, kind of like the deductible on your car insurance, during which you pay for the full cost of care before your coverage kicks in. Elimination periods typically range from twenty days to over one hundred, and the shorter the time frame the higher the premium. My father's policy didn't have much in the way of bells and whistles, but we were glad he had one at all. As his need for care intensified, it certainly came in handy.

Adult Day Care: The Price Is Right

During the first few years of my father's dementia, we never considered a nursing home. Bubbie's four-year stint in a home with long hours tied to a chair had left a bad taste in our mouths. How could we possibly put my father in a place like that? As the disease progressed, we knew there might come a day when my mother could no longer handle my father's care. So we explored supports that would give my mom a break and provide my father with some variety to his day. We landed on adult day care, a cost-effective and often overlooked option for care. At an average daily cost of $68, it's a bargain.[13] Adult day care offers flexibility and support in a community-based setting. Some programs, like the one my father attended, are specifically designed for people with dementia and Alzheimer's disease. My dad enjoyed the sing-alongs and exercise program (okay, he played catch with a beach ball while sitting in a wheelchair, but he loved it!). My mom drove him to the program several times a week (transportation was extra). And my father looked forward to the change in venue while my mother had some time for herself. Meanwhile, my dad's long-term care insurance policy had kicked in to cover the cost of adult day care. But our biggest looming worry was nursing home care—a costly option that might be needed down the road.

It Costs How Much? Nursing Homes and Assisted Living

There was no dramatic event that made us realize things needed to change. Instead, it was the unrelenting disease progression with its slew of losses that chipped away at my father's last hold on independence. My mother was growing weary and my father was slipping away. Making the decision to put a loved one in a nursing home can be agonizing. Many families prefer the option of assisted living, which is less stigmatizing and offers more independence than a nursing home. Comparing the cost of assisted living to nursing homes is like comparing apples to oranges as the two types of institutions provide very different levels of care. The national median rate for assisted living is $3,628 per month, or $43,500 per year.[14] Sounds like a bargain compared to nursing homes. Perhaps it is, but not necessarily. Room and board, along with some meals, are typically included in the monthly fee. If your mother needs a home health aide, however, it may be costly because nonmedical home care is usually not covered in the monthly fee. If you run out of money, don't expect Medicaid to kick in since most assisted living communities don't accept it. (Some do under state Medicaid waiver programs, but you can't count on it.) Long-term care insurance may cover assisted living; it depends on the policy. Once you start using your long-term care insurance benefit, you no longer pay premiums, so there's a little savings there.

Before my father could use his long-term care insurance, he first had to qualify under the policy guidelines and be unable to perform at least two activities of daily living (such as bathing, dressing, eating, and going to the bathroom). My father passed that test with flying colors. He could no longer walk, and although he could still feed himself, he needed help with all other activities of daily living. We were resigned to the necessity of going the nursing home route. My father's graceful acceptance of this transition was an unexpected gift that eased our guilt. My knowledge of the long-term care system eliminated much of the guesswork but not the challenges to come. The nursing home we chose had many positives. It had a warm and inviting atmosphere and the smell of fresh-baked cookies filled the air. Cats and birds were counted among the full-time residents, and it was only a fifteen-minute drive from my mother's home. As nursing homes went, it was better than acceptable. At a cost of $90,000 per year, the long-term care insurance came in handy and allowed my mother to afford the hefty price tag—for a while.

Nobody likes to think about shelling out life savings for a nursing home. They are expensive enterprises for a good reason. Unlike assisted living communities, nursing homes provide twenty-four-hour nursing and medical care for people with chronic illness and dementia, like my dad. The median annual cost of a nursing home is about $82,000, but can vary significantly depending on where you live. If your parent lives in the great state of Texas you're in luck, at least when it comes to nursing home costs. At about $52,000 a year, the Lone Star State is a bargain compared to nursing homes in Alaska, where the median price tag is just under $300,000.[15] Private rooms are preferable for some folks, but you'll pay about $10,000 less a year for a "semi-private" room. My father always shared a room and didn't seem to mind the arrangement. One of my dad's roommates was a resident who bellowed loudly throughout the day, despite efforts by the nursing staff to calm him down. I asked my father if he minded the noise. "No," he replied. "It's kind of entertaining." In my father's case, sharing a room meant having company. Despite the cacophony, it worked for him, but he may be the exception. The extra cost for a private room might be worth it if it gives your parent the privacy he needs or makes her more comfortable

A Place to Age in Place

Once my father moved to a nursing home, the big old house we grew up in felt empty. It required more upkeep than my mother could handle and was not senior friendly. My mother, emotionally attached to the home where she had lived for fifty-plus years, was initially reluctant to move, but after she broke her elbow from tripping on the stairs, she realized it was time for a change. My folks could have benefited from a continuing care retirement community (CCRC), also known as a life care community. These multilevel communities allow people to age in place by offering a combination of living arrangements along a continuum: from independent to assisted living to nursing home level of care. Residents typically enter as independent and may be required to pay a substantial entry fee—a portion of which may be refunded to their estate upon death. Entrance fees vary widely and typically mirror the real estate market. CCRCs in the Boston area, a real estate hotspot, have significantly higher entrance fees—they can exceed $1 million! And that's just to get in. Monthly fees average around $3,000 and vary significantly depending on the type of contract, location, services, and level of care. It's enough to make your head spin. Aging life care professionals can provide expert advice on which CCRCs to consider given your family's situation. Attorneys also should be consulted when sorting through the various CCRC contracts and plans so they can explain what you're getting into.

About a year after my father moved to the nursing home, my mother began exploring senior housing options that would allow her to remain independent but still have access to care if she needed it. At the time, there were few CCRCs in western Massachusetts. So instead, my mother opted for a retirement community that had assisted living on its campus, euphemistically referred to as "the Inn"—kind of like a CCRC without the nursing home. My mother hired a senior move manager, a professional who helps seniors and their families with the daunting task of downsizing and relocation. I don't know how my mother would ever have moved without her. My mom had saved everything from her children's preschool drawings to high school essays, so there was a lot of stuff to sort through. But the move manager made it all happen. Furniture was sold or given away, clutter was unceremoniously tossed, and precious memorabilia were sorted and saved. With the sale of the house, my mother was able to afford a lovely two-bedroom, one-story townhouse within an idyllic retirement community. She now has neighbors who are friends and a built-in safety net should she need care. To describe my mother as happy in this community is an understatement. And my dad was in a nursing home nearby, allowing her to visit him every day.

Being a Veteran Can Pay Off

My father spent three years in the nursing home with the cats and the cookies. Other than eating too many sweets and gaining too much weight, he generally fared well. My mother knew his long-term care insurance would eventually run out, but my father was not eligible for Medicaid either. Between my father's pension and his long-term care insurance, my mother had enough money to last a few years. Beyond that, we needed a new plan. As a U.S. Army veteran, my father was eligible for benefits, something we had not previously considered. The VA.gov website has a lot of valuable information about long-term care, including disability compensation, residential programs, and the aid and attendance benefit, which increases the pension amount for homebound veterans. There's a lot of stuff to sort through and it can be overwhelming. Veterans Financial (www.veteransfinancial.com), a national company specializing in veterans' financial services, helped with the daunting task of figuring out eligibility and documentation requirements. While it was a bit of a slog, with lots of paperwork—like digging up my dad's military discharge records—it paid off. We put my father on a two-year waiting list for the Soldiers' Home, a state-run facility that cares for disabled veterans. After just one year we got the call. A bed was ready at the Soldiers' Home, and we had forty-eight hours to move my father. Transitioning my father from a nursing home where he was happy and well cared for was a difficult and agonizing decision. But the difference in cost was substantial—$9,000 a month for the private pay home versus $900 a month at the veterans' facility. Did my dad get good care at the Soldiers' Home? Yes—for the most part he did. Was it perfect? No—it never is. But he spent three years there and seemed content. Several months after the move, I asked my father to rate the Soldiers' Home on a scale of one to ten (Ritz Carlton versus crappy motel again). He rated it an eight. "Eight," I said. "That's pretty good. Why not higher?" "Well, there's always room for improvement," responded my dad wisely.

Part of the reason my father fared so well was that my mother was an extraordinary advocate. She was at the nursing home every day, rain or shine, and was in constant contact with the staff about my father's care. Visiting regularly and communicating with the team of nurses, aides, and physicians generally translates to better care. Being an effective caregiver advocate takes patience, communication skills, and some basic understanding of the healthcare system.

In the next chapter, you'll learn how to navigate the byzantine world of long-term care. Knowing what care costs is a good first step. But finding care that is accessible, affordable, and acceptable to your parent is another challenge entirely. The healthcare system doesn't make it easy. You may feel like you have entered a strange world where the hospital, nursing home, and home care agency speak in tongues. Shouldn't all our modern technology provide for better communication across different types of care? That is the goal. Now prepare yourself for the reality.

SIX

The Care Maze

America's health care system is neither healthy,
caring, nor a system.
—WALTER CRONKITE

Our healthcare system, designed to heal and comfort, can feel inhospitable and daunting to seniors and their families as they try to navigate this fragmented and complex world. Many people find themselves thrust into a caregiving role after their father suffers a stroke or their mother is diagnosed with stage-four breast cancer. Suddenly you are riding an un-merry-go-round, bouncing from doctors' offices, emergency rooms, and hospitals to home—like a never-ending loop. You may be forced to make hasty decisions, without adequate preparation or guidance, leading to the next crisis du jour. You desperately want to communicate with the healthcare team, but it's hard to know whom you should talk to about what. The doctors, nurses, and social workers are highly trained professionals who are trying to work within a system that doesn't necessarily work for them—or their patients. I should know. I was one of them.

I started my social work career in the early 1980s, first as a master's-level social work intern and later as a staff social worker at the MGH (Massachusetts General Hospital) in Boston. There, I not only landed my first job, I also found my husband—a psychiatrist completing his residency training at the time. After seven years of being a small fish in a very big pond, I decided to leave MGH. When I jumped ship to work at a nearby community hospital, the reaction among my colleagues was incredulous. What could I possibly gain from leaving one of the best hospitals in the world and going to a *community* (code word for "backward") hospital instead? Answer: a lot.

I spent the next five years as a director of social service and utilization review in a hospital just north of Boston that had one of the highest geriatric populations in the state. I oversaw a team of dedicated social workers and nurses who worked with patients and their families to come up with a sound plan of discharge. We started this process by meeting with patients shortly after their admission to the hospital. Many were discharged with home care, some were transferred to rehab facilities, and those who could no longer live independently were often sent to nursing homes. We worked closely with patients and families to teach them about the discharge process upfront so they would not be caught off guard. We visited area nursing homes to get the inside scoop on each facility. And we made sure that information was effectively communicated among the healthcare team so that discharge went as smoothly as possible.

Overall, it was a wonderful opportunity to be part of an expanding network of care that focused on the needs of seniors and their families. The hospital built a nursing home on its campus with a state-of-the-art Alzheimer's unit. For complex medical and psychiatric conditions, the hospital had a "geri-psych" unit where elderly patients received specialized treatment and monitoring. There was also a sub-acute rehabilitation unit so people recovering from hip fractures and strokes could be transferred within the hospital for rehab, rather than to an outside facility. Later, a hospital-based home health agency was added to provide continuity of care for patients being discharged back to the community. This little hospital, under the shadow of the big teaching hospitals, was the little engine that could. We were pushing the envelope of traditional, more siloed healthcare by creating a continuum of care under one umbrella. Professionally, it was an exciting time for me. It was also eye-opening. I learned a lot about what can go wrong when patients move from one level of care to another. And I saw how families struggled to make plans for their loved ones when they had just days to make life-altering decisions.

Beware of Hospitals

A friend of mine, who recently turned sixty, came down with a sudden and nasty bacterial infection of the skin. After running a 5k, she felt sluggish and clammy, which she initially attributed to the effects of exertion. When a strange red blotch appeared on her leg and her temperature spiked to 104 degrees, she became concerned. After a trip to the ER, my friend was admitted to her local hospital and spent several days on IV antibiotics. By the third day, she felt much better. "It was a lousy experience," she said. "But I got great care." One of the reasons our life expectancy has increased so dramatically is that hospitals, like the one where my friend was treated, save lives. Whether you are in a car accident, suffer a stroke, or have a heart attack, the place you want to be is a good-quality hospital with top-notch care. But for a frail, older person, hospitals can be a dangerous place. An elder's immune system may already be compromised, making them vulnerable to hospital-acquired infections. These "nosocomial infections," as they are called, can spread like the infamous norovirus on a cruise ship—without the fun of ever having been at sea. Lying in a hospital bed all day just isn't good for you and can lead to weak muscles and festering bed sores. Those with dementia, like my dad, may become even more confused from the harsh lights and constant buzz of activity that come with the territory. And don't expect Marcus Welby at your bedside. The doctor who oversees your care is probably a "hospitalist," a physician specializing in hospital care, who doesn't know you personally.

Put the Plan Back in Discharge Planning

The moment you get admitted to the hospital, the clock starts ticking. I was once that friendly discharge planner whose job was to plan your departure from the hospital soon after you arrived. Why is it so important to start this process right away? To begin with, hospitals have a big incentive to keep a patient's length of stay as short as possible. Under Medicare, a hospital is paid a fixed amount of money, based largely on a patient's diagnosis. When I oversaw utilization review, a system of monitoring the necessity and efficiency of medical services, a nurse on my team had to make sure that patients occupying a bed were considered "hospital level of care." If a patient didn't medically need to be in the hospital anymore, the nurse would urge the patient's doctor to sign a discharge order. Families were given forty-eight hours—or less—to make a decision about their loved one's care—which was not always enough time to get it right.

A Crash Course in Caregiving

At thirty-three, life was going well for Derek. He'd recently landed a coveted job at an e-commerce company. His long-term girlfriend had accepted his marriage proposal. After purchasing a condo, Derek felt he was embracing life as a full-fledged grown-up. Then one day his sister Marcella called. Derek's father Tony had suffered stroke-like symptoms and had been rushed to the hospital. Derek dropped everything and met his sister in the emergency room, where they spent seven long hours waiting for their father to be admitted. Little did they know that this was the start of a two-year odyssey that would leave them frustrated and depleted. As young adults, just launching their personal and professional lives, caregiving was not something they had planned for or anticipated. Their father was only in his late sixties and despite a few idiosyncrasies, he had seemed okay. Or so they thought.

Looking back, there were signs they had missed. Derek's dad had appeared more anxious and reclusive since his divorce from Derek's mother. He preferred to meet in neutral places and never invited Derek and Marcella to his apartment. Although Tony had never been a laid-back guy, he seemed increasingly worried about everyday activities like driving and going to the bathroom. Once Derek and his sister understood what was going on, things started adding up. They found out from the doctors at the hospital that Tony had suffered a brain bleed; he was also diagnosed with early-stage dementia. But after only three days in the hospital, he was discharged home. Derek and Marcella realized their father's situation was worse than they had thought. When they took Tony home, they were shocked at the condition of his apartment. Newspapers, some of which were months old, were strewn everywhere. Old food was rotting in the fridge. Mounds of dirty laundry carpeted the place. Derek and Marcella learned that Tony had been hoarding, an irrational and persistent need to hold on to things. Hoarding earned its own stand-alone category in the American Psychiatric Association standard reference work, the *Diagnostic and Statistical Manual of Mental Disorders*, fifth edition (*DSM-5*), updated in

2013. It is a difficult condition to treat. As the hoarder continues to accumulate stuff, there may be more clutter than living space. Even Tony's bed was covered with boxes and garbage bags. Hoarding can also be a warning sign of cognitive impairment and dementia among seniors. Derek and Marcella came to the grim realization that their father was declining fast and needed specialized care. At the time, getting him the right care—and finding a way to pay for it—seemed like a daunting task.

After his discharge home, it wasn't long before Tony became so anxious and confused that he called 911. He was sent back to the hospital and then transferred to a geriatric psychiatric unit for evaluation and treatment. He was put on medication that made him less anxious but more lethargic. He was taught behavioral techniques to quell his fears and compulsive thoughts. Just days before discharge, a social worker met with Derek and Marcella and suggested assisted living, with a price tag of over $6,000 a month. "My dad didn't have that kind of money and neither did we," Derek recalls. "The discharge planner didn't even discuss costs. She made recommendations that were way out of our reach." At the time, Tony did not have Medicaid, so the options for long-term care were limited. The complexity of Tony's mental health needs, in addition to dementia, made the situation even harder. He was sent home with written instructions about care, which he was unable to follow. His condition deteriorated, and it was not long before Tony ended up in a hospital once again.

The next two years were a series of trial and error, with the emphasis on error. Tony had a brief stay in affordable senior housing after being on a waiting list for nine months. While the price was right, the setting was wrong. When alone Tony would panic, usually about eating, choking, or going to the bathroom, and call his kids or 911 for help. Tony needed more support than either Derek or Marcella could provide. He was hospitalized several more times, but the focus was always on short-term treatment instead of a long-term sustainable plan. Eventually Derek learned of an eldercare benefit through work that helped employees like him. He now had access to a care advisor to guide him and his sister through the uncharted terrain of senior care. The advisor helped Derek get Tony on Mass Health (Massachusetts Medicaid), which expanded their options for long-term care. In addition, the advisor identified a nursing home that could manage Tony's medical and psychiatric care needs and accepted Medicaid. "The system is really broken," explained Derek. "My sister and I were throwing darts at a target without a bull's-eye. We had no idea what we were doing. Unfortunately, the healthcare system wasn't much help. Over the last two years, I got married, became a dad, and put my father in a nursing home. That's a real crash course in becoming a grown-up."

Frequent Flyers

Patients like Tony who bounce in and out of hospitals are the focus of a lot of attention in healthcare these days—for good reason. These unfortunate frequent flyers, many of whom are readmitted to the hospital within thirty days of discharge, make up one-fifth of all Medicare beneficiaries and cost $26 billion annually.[1] More than half of these readmissions are considered preventable. Family caregivers like Derek and Marcella play a critical role in transitioning their loved ones from hospital to home or some other type of care. All too often, family members are ignored, dismissed, or not sufficiently engaged. Dr. Robert L. Kane, a nationally respected geriatrician and author of over twenty-five books on long-term care, describes our current discharge system as a national disgrace. Kane does not mince words when it comes to discharge planners. "Think of them the way you would a salesperson," he says. "In their eyes, the first train leaving the station is the best one to get the older patient on, even if it is not going where the patient wants."[2]

As Derek learned the hard way, the transition from hospital to home does not always go smoothly. When it doesn't, people like Tony may bounce back to the hospital or decline further at home. Why is that? A lot of information gets communicated at discharge: appointments need to be scheduled, prescriptions filled, home care reviewed—and that's just for starters. Discharge summaries, those handy-dandy sets of instructions that are important to read and comprehend, may not be clearly explained to the patient and family. All too often, family caregivers are left to figure out complex medical instructions on their own and to assume the role of de facto nurse when they've had absolutely no medical training. When it comes to managing wound care and IVs, your high school biology course thirty years ago just doesn't cut it.

Florence Nightingale, Where Are You?

Back in the mid-1990s, when I ran a home health care agency, it was the visiting nurse who managed a patient's medical needs and the family who helped with household chores and personal care. But with shorter hospital stays and advances in technology, families are now assuming another role when their loved one goes home from the hospital—Florence Nightingale—just without the training or iconic status. The *Home Alone* study, conducted by

AARP and the United Hospital Fund, found close to half of family caregivers perform in-home medical and nursing tasks for their family members with multiple chronic and cognitive conditions.[3] They—mostly daughters—are managing medication, administering enemas, operating feeding tubes, and tending to wounds. Many find the dual role of devoted daughter and attentive nursemaid physically and emotionally taxing. Some take solace in the fact that they are playing an important role in keeping their parent alive—or at least out of a nursing home. At the same time, performing multiple medical tasks can pose risks to the caregiver and lead to increased stress and depression.[4] Families take on this responsibility for a mixture of reasons: devotion, love, guilt, and the belief that they have little choice in the matter. It's as if there is a silent contract between the healthcare system and the family. Your mother's coming home. Tag, you're it—ready or not.

A Step in the Right Direction

Viewing the family caregiver as an essential part of the hospital discharge plan seems like a no-brainer. Many families may not fully understand what discharge planning is all about. The "discharge" part becomes all too evident when they get a call that their father's going home from the hospital. But the planning piece? Not so much. This is what should happen: the designated family caregiver's name should be recorded at the time of a patient's hospital admission, adequate notice should be given prior to discharge, and comprehensible instructions on home care tasks, especially medically related ones, should be provided (and demonstrated) before the patient leaves the hospital. These best practices may be common in some hospitals, but not in others. Now, following these practices is not only a good idea: it is the law in a growing number of states. In 2014, AARP proposed the CARE (Caregiver Advise, Record, and Enable) Act so that family members like Derek are not left in the lurch when their loved one gets discharged.[5]

There are also encouraging trends to address the needs of frail seniors, especially those without adequate family or community support, many of whom have both Medicare and Medicaid. Coined the "dual eligibles," these people are some of the sickest, poorest, and costliest patients to care for. The good news is that programs are springing up around the country to better understand and address the needs of this vulnerable population. These community transition programs, funded by hospitals as well as state and federal grants, offer a wide range of services such as case management, in-home care, and transportation. The goal is to provide much-needed community support to frail elders who are at risk for bouncing back to the hospital after discharge. Sometimes the reasons for preventable readmission are pretty basic. Your mother doesn't have a ride to the doctor for a follow-up appointment or she gets her meds mixed up. Perhaps your dad has to stick with a salt-free diet and his cupboards are stocked with peanuts and potato chips. Or maybe he is alone in an unsafe apartment, like Derek's father, and needs more oversight. Solving these problems drives down costs, improves care, and just makes sense. Your local Area Agency on Aging can clue you in to programs in your area, along with eligibility requirements. Some programs are short-term and focus on the thirty days after discharge, when patients are most likely to get readmitted. That's also the same period of time when hospitals may pay a hefty penalty if they do.

Pushing Back

The discharge process may be fraught with land mines, but what do you do when the time frame just doesn't make sense—like being given twenty-four hours to choose a nursing home for your mother in Poughkeepsie—and you live in Los Angeles? Or your father with early-stage dementia is being discharged home—alone—with a sheet of instructions he can't understand. You are not Houdini.

You can't magically appear or get yourself out of a bind without speaking up. You and your parent are entitled to a reasonable amount of time to make life-altering plans for post-hospital care. While there may be some disagreement about what "reasonable" means, you may be able to buy some time if you push back on what you think is an unsafe plan. Even a day or two may help when it comes to making big decisions about care and finding the right provider. Meanwhile, pay attention to your parent's rights under Medicare. Within two days of your mother's admission to the hospital, she will receive a written notice that says: "Important Message from Medicare."[6] Included in this notice is a Medicare bill of rights, so don't toss it out with the Kleenex on the counter. If the hospital's pressuring your mom to go, but you don't think it's safe, your bill of rights will explain the appeal process. It is not something to undertake lightly, but it's good to know about if other measures fail.

Do Your Research

While it goes against human nature to cram for a crisis before it occurs, a little preparation can go a long way. Exploring options ahead of time may give you a better idea of the lay of the land if you need to choose an assisted living community or nursing home on short notice. But where do you begin? The list of providers the discharge planner hands you is not much to go on. Does assisted living make sense if your parent is going to need more care down the road? And how do you tell which nursing homes will provide the best care and which ones to avoid at all costs?

One of the toughest decisions to make under the gun is choosing the right nursing home. As a discharge planner, I saw families make this emotionally wrenching choice on a Wednesday because their father was being discharged on a Thursday. As my dad once said, "That is no way to run a railroad." It takes time, research, and a village to get it right. The discharge planner will give you a list of facilities to choose from. That's a start. Seek recommendations from friends, neighbors, and healthcare providers familiar with local long-term care options. If you can afford it, you may want to hire an aging life care professional. Employers can also be a good resource and are increasingly offering support to their caregiving employees like Derek. If you are in the workplace, reach out to your manager or human resource department and find out if your organization has an employer-supported eldercare program.

Your village should also include your local long-term care ombudsman. Directed by the Administration on Aging (AoA), ombudsmen resolve problems between families and long-term care facilities and can instruct you about residents' rights. An ombudsman probably won't tell you which provider to choose, but can steer you away from facilities that have a history of complaints from families and residents. Keep in mind that ombudsmen are mostly volunteers and some are more informative and knowledgeable than others. It's a free service and you can find an ombudsman by going to ltcombudsman.org.

It's Not the Fountain in the Lobby

In April 2006, I made a visit to western Massachusetts with the specific intent of finding a nursing home for my father. Most visits to my hometown were spent shopping at hip boutiques and eating farm-to-table food at cafés filled with college students. This time I came with a more solemn purpose. I was going to support my mother through one of the toughest decisions of her life. Some families refuse to consider a nursing home altogether because they see it as "dumping" their loved one in an institution. This belief is particularly strong in certain cultures where nursing home care is associated with a great deal of stigma, guilt, and shame.

While the decision was not guilt-free for me and my family, we knew it was the right thing to do. Together, we would determine where my father would spend the remaining years of his life: a place where he would hopefully be comfortable, well cared for, and content. I came prepared with information about five nursing homes in the area, some of which had attractive lobbies and inviting dining rooms. Others looked tired and in need of a coat of paint—or two. I tried to assure my mother that the fountain in the lobby isn't going to matter one whit to Dad. She was not easily convinced.

Our mission was to find a place that didn't just warehouse residents but would care for their bodies *and* their souls. That meant looking beyond the obvious to what was most important: a culture of caring. I made appointments with administrators in each of the five facilities and brought a copy of their last state inspection survey results, including any deficiencies that had been cited. Some looked at me like I had two heads; others seemed defensive. Although I took the survey into account, I also focused on how the administrator responded to my numerous questions. That would be an important indicator of how problems would be addressed down the road.

It may be a small measure of comfort to know that the nursing home industry is one of the most regulated in America, second only to nuclear power. There are over 130,000 pages of federal regulations that govern nursing facilities, but I don't recommend you add them to your summer reading list. Fortunately, you can get easy access, as I did, to the web-based Nursing Home Compare rating system (www.medicare.gov/nursinghomecompare) developed by the Centers for Medicare and Medicaid Services (CMS). Nursing homes undergo annual inspections that address a wide range of issues, including quality of care practices, medication administration, and fire safety. There is lots of data here so don't get lost in the weeds. Reviewing health inspection results, staffing ratios, and facility maintenance will give you a snapshot of how nursing homes compare to one another and which ones have a pattern of serious violations. Keep in mind that not all deficiencies carry the same weight; some are more egregious than others. You may want someone familiar with the survey process to help interpret the data in a balanced and meaningful way. When visiting a nursing home, don't be afraid to ask about deficiencies and find out what has been done to correct them.

The nursing home we ultimately chose for my father had a survey report that was far from glowing. There were numerous deficiencies, and the overall rating fell below average. I would have crossed that facility off the list entirely, but it was my mother's first choice. Her friend had recommended the place and it was close to home, an important consideration given that my mother planned to visit every day. When we met with the nursing home administrator, I discovered she'd been in her position for over five years. That was a good sign since excessive turnover can indicate instability within nursing homes. I also brought up the inspection survey results and her response impressed me. She not only acknowledged the deficiencies, she showed me the corrective action plan she'd submitted to the state. After the last survey, the nursing home had implemented a training program for direct care staff to be more responsive to the residents, especially in the dementia unit. That got my attention. And the most recent inspection report showed no deficiencies at all. While that information was useful, it was just one data point. You need to dig deeper and conduct your own survey of sorts. But first you need to know what to look for and how to find it.

Use Your Senses

The best tools at your disposal are your own senses, including the most important one—your common sense. Schedule a visit and look around. Are residents lined up unattended in the corridors, lethargic and moaning? Or are they plunked in front of the TV while an aide sits passively reading the paper? Take a whiff. If the place smells of bodily fluids or disinfectant, that's not a good sign.

Observe. Are the staff members chatting at the nurse's station while ignoring the residents' calls? Yes, these are all things I have seen in nursing homes—repeatedly. No wonder these places get such a bad rap. But I have also uncovered what's good about them. Certified nursing assistants like Roseline, whose soft touch and loving nature elicited my father's warm, appreciative smile and air kisses. Or the activities director who went beyond bingo and started a nursing home chorus, composed mostly of residents belting out show tunes. And the nurse who referred to my father as "Professor" and understood that the quiet man slumped over in his wheelchair still had a big heart and an active mind.

Another way to conduct your own survey is to do what I did: perch yourself in the nursing home lobby (hopefully without a fountain) and talk with visiting family members at random. Some may not want to chat, but most will. They'll give you the lowdown and share their observations, both good and bad. You may need to take their comments with a grain of salt, but your data-gathering can give you important insight from people who really know the place. Most important, visit the facility more than once, and not just under the guided tour of the admissions director. Stop by during a shift change or on the weekend. No matter what nursing home you choose, it's important that someone checks in on your loved one often and gets to know the staff. Residents whose family members visit regularly tend to fare better overall.

Ask about the "Assist" in Assisted Living

If your mother can't manage to live alone anymore but doesn't need 24/7 care, assisted living might be a good option. Assisted living facilities (ALFs) were initially designed as an alternative to nursing homes for folks who needed some assistance but were generally pretty independent. Over the past thirty-five years, assisted living has evolved to include a broad range of things. It might be a quaint little apartment with access to meals and a built-in community or care for your parent with late-stage dementia. Assisted living is less institutional than a nursing home and tends to look more like a hotel (with nursing staff) than a healthcare facility.

Unlike nursing homes, which are heavily regulated, ALFs exist under varying state oversight or the lack thereof. That makes it harder to gather data that can help you compare one assisted living community to another. When you go for a visit, you will likely be given a tour by an enthusiastic marketing director who will tell you what you want to hear. Come prepared with the right questions so you can look beyond the sales pitch. What is included in the monthly fee and what is extra? Can you hire your own paid caregiver or do you need to use a designated home care agency? How are the medical needs of the residents addressed? Are there types of care the assisted living community *cannot* manage? If your mother's dementia progresses or if she becomes aggressive, will she need to leave? Knowing that ahead of time may save you a lot of grief and guesswork.

Be an Advocate

Whatever care your mother ultimately requires, whether it is a nursing home, assisted living, or home care, she will need an advocate. If you are reading this book, chances are that person is you. Where do you start? Many caregivers begin this journey in the doctor's office. While you may feel comfortable questioning your doctor or asking for a second opinion, your mother may not. I've been seeing my gynecologist for thirty years and I call her Sharon. I don't hold back when addressing concerns about my health. AARP found that people actively involved in managing their illnesses have better outcomes.[7] But if your mother isn't comfortable or willing to speak up, you might need to be her voice.

Dr. Susan Weinstein, an internist with a large geriatric practice, recommends that families plan ahead for the visit. She suggests you bring along lists of medications, healthcare questions, observations or concerns about driving. "And bring up the most important questions at the beginning of the session," says Weinstein. "If there is a laundry list of issues we may not get to them all." Weinstein also recommends that families find a way to communicate with each other and share information either in a single notebook or securely online. "When there are a number of family members with different perspectives, it can make it harder to agree on the right plan of care."

If you are the chief family caregiver and advocate, you should also get a signed HIPAA release, which gives you access to your parent's medical information under the Health Insurance Portability and Accountability Act and allows you to communicate with your parent's doctor more freely. HIPAA regulations are designed to protect patient privacy, but if they are too rigidly interpreted by healthcare professionals, they could serve as a barrier between you and your parent's physician. To make matters more confusing, there is no standard HIPAA form, and doctors, hospitals, and healthcare providers often require you use their version. Without one, you may not get information when it's most needed.

Attention Must Be Paid

As caregivers, we try our best to navigate the health-care system and make sure our parent's voice is heard. After my mother's femur fracture, I accompanied her to monthly follow-up appointments to the orthopedist—as her daughter and advocate. But as soon as we checked in at the reception desk there was a problem. The receptionist spoke to me as if my mother, looking straight at her from a wheelchair, was invisible. My mother stared at her and said, "I am right here. I can hear and I can speak. Please talk directly to me." Go, Mom!

All too often, we dismiss, ignore, or patronize our elders. This happens in families and within the healthcare system. It happens in doctor's offices and in hospitals. While "patient-centered" healthcare is considered a new and evolving trend, it should be a given. That said, we cannot assume things will go smoothly. Attention must be paid—we are our parents' keepers. We help them get the care they need and make sure their needs are heard.

We would want nothing less for ourselves.

SEVEN

Making Work Work

Balance is not about better time management, but about
better boundary management. Balance means making
choices and enjoying those choices.
—BETSY JACOBSON, WORK AND LIFE BALANCE COACH

Sometimes when it comes to work/life balance I feel like
I missed the boat. Yes, I somehow balanced it all—kids,
my career, and caring for my dad. Back then there was no
open forum, like Facebook or blogs, to describe all the
madness and get some support. When it came to work
and caregiving, I often felt alone. The best thing to do
as a working caregiver, or so I thought, was just to show
up and shut up. But there's only so long you can keep
the caregiving side of your life hidden at work. Sooner or

later, life intrudes and you are exposed for who you truly are: a caregiver.

When I returned to work after my third child was born, I was determined to continue nursing and feed my daughter breast milk rather than formula. That meant I had to pump at work, using a contraption the size of a carry-on suitcase. This was 1993, many years before employers were required to provide break time for mothers to express milk and a private place to do so. So I took the bigger-than-a-breadbox breast pump to the only place I could get some privacy: the ladies' room. There I sat on the toilet trying my darnedest to express eight ounces of milk for my little munchkin back home. After an hour of great effort, I got enough for a few gulps. And then I spilled it—all over the bathroom floor. As contrived as it may sound, I *did* cry over spilt milk. But there was much more to my distress than that.

Fast-forward ten years. I have three school-aged kids and a father with dementia, who is living with me during my mother's recovery from hip surgery. I was a sandwich-generation caregiver, caring for both my parents and children, before that was something people talked about. By then, parenthood had caught the attention of employers. Many had introduced workplace benefits so that raising children and having a job would be less of a dizzying tightrope walk. That was a step in the right direction. But employer-supported eldercare, addressing the needs of employees caring for aging parents and family members, was still in the dark ages.

No Backup Plan

> Good morning, Dad. Mom's in the hospital. She's had a hip replacement and she's okay. We are going to visit her today.

I wrote those words on a big manila sign that I hung in my kitchen so my father could see it every morning as he was having breakfast. It prevented my dad from worrying unnecessarily about my mother's absence and provided reassurance that she was fine. During the hours I was at work, I hired a paid caregiver to keep an eye on my father until I came home. Then I would pick Dad up and we'd head over to the hospital to visit my mother. We had a predictable routine in place and it was working—until it wasn't. One day the caregiver didn't show up and I had no backup plan. I was scheduled to attend an important meeting so I needed to think fast. "Dad," I said, "how'd you like to come to work with me today?" "Sure," he answered agreeably. It was not Take Your Dad with Dementia to Work Day. But I brought him anyway.

Although it worked out—sort of—I don't recommend taking your parent to work as a backup plan. But that experience got me thinking. There must be a better way to manage the inevitable disruptions in care that prevent you from getting your job done or showing up at all. So I decided to refocus my career to help solve this problem. I created an adult backup care program within a company that provided short-term, on-demand child and senior care. Years later, I created an eldercare program to support working caregivers, which became part of Care.com's suite of employer benefits across the life span. Over the past decade, I've helped people juggle their work and family responsibilities, and I know what they're up against. Without enough support, these folks will struggle on all fronts. If they fail, *everyone*—including the employee, employer, and the family member needing care—will pay a price.

The day I brought my father to work I remember thinking, "I can't be the only person dealing with this stuff. There must be other working stiffs caring for their parents and making it up us as they go." In fact, 60 percent of the nation's 40 million unpaid family caregivers are employed full- or part-time. Of these, one in four is a millennial.[1] There are a lot of us in this boat. And many are struggling to stay focused on the job while making sure Mom or Dad is okay. If you're one of them, chances are you've arrived late to work because you took your mother to the doctor. Or you missed a client meeting because the caregiver didn't show up. Maybe you're googling "home care" when you should be finalizing your Q3 goals. And the fear of getting "the call" is always in the back of your mind, because you know you're just one crisis away from it all falling down like a house of cards.

If you are dealing with senior care challenges at work and trying to act like everything is okay, forget about it. Close to 70 percent of working caregivers experience work-related disruptions due to their dual roles, and it's not something you can easily hide.[2] When the going gets too tough, some quit their jobs altogether. But there's often a heavy cost for those who do. Over a lifetime, employees who leave the workforce to care for a parent lose close to $300,000 in wages and benefits, and the amount is even higher for women.[3] So if you are a working caregiver, what do you do to stay in the game? While you do your best to show up, too much shutting up may make things worse. That means you'll have to speak up, ask for what you need, and learn to be your own best advocate.

The Long-Distance Working Caregiver

Under the best of circumstances, the life of a salesperson has its ups and downs. At forty-eight, Phil had twenty years of sales experience. His job selling analytics to financial services companies was an exciting but high-pressure position. He'd always been a top performer, but year-end quotas combined with longer than anticipated sales cycles weighed him down. A new thirty-something boss routinely sent texts and emails late at night and on weekends, expecting his team to always be on. Phil did his best to respond quickly and meet his goals. He was counting on those fat commissions to make some much-needed repairs to his home. What he wasn't counting on was an eldercare crisis.

Phil's parents, both in their eighties, had managed to live pretty independently despite a few setbacks now and then. Their home was in a small town called Shiner, Texas. It didn't help that Phil lived almost fifteen hundred miles away in Pittsburgh. Regular phone calls and the occasional visit to Shiner was all he could fit into his busy schedule. But as his father's Parkinson's disease worsened, the minor setbacks morphed into major problems. Phil's mother, all five feet of her, could not handle the heavy lifting required to get her husband out of bed in the morning. But that didn't stop her from trying. Like many spousal caregivers, Phil's mother was at risk for injuring herself. One day when she was caring for Phil's dad, she did just that and ruptured a disc. There was no longer any debate:

Mom's lifting days were over. Now it was up to Phil to figure out what to do next. And he felt pretty alone with all the responsibility. Recently divorced, Phil had a brother who lived abroad and checked in through email, but that was it.

Suddenly, Phil found himself in a club with a growing membership—family caregivers in the workforce. Unlike the majority of employed caregivers, who are women, Phil was a man in a male-dominated field. He had no intention of sharing his family saga with his text-happy always-on boss. Meanwhile, Phil was taking time off to shuttle back and forth to Texas to figure out how best to help his parents. Those missed days started to add up and draw unwanted attention. On average, working caregivers miss six and a half days of work a year.[4] Like Phil, they are stressed out, distracted, or simply not able to focus on their jobs. In addition to the missed days, Phil's work started to suffer. His sales numbers dropped and his hope for commissions evaporated. Emails sat unanswered in his inbox. Phil knew he was barely treading water but dared not speak up. "I didn't leave my job, but in some sense I did. I was stalled out and exhausted. I lived with a constant fear of failure. Failing at my job, failing to meet my expenses, and worst of all, failing to take care of my parents."

Little Shiner, Texas, may be home to a one-hundred-year-old brewery, but it's not exactly a haven for eldercare.

In addition, the long-distance caregiving was taking a toll and certainly not helping Phil close any deals. Caregivers who live a distance from their loved ones face additional hardships: they struggle to find and coordinate care and often report higher levels of stress than caregivers on the scene. Phil eventually came to the conclusion that the situation was unsustainable. He needed to convince his parents to move to Pittsburgh so they could live closer to him. But first he had to begin the process of finding them a suitable living arrangement—something that would take lots of time he didn't have.

While Phil was committed to his job, he had to re-balance his priorities, at least in the short run. He was going to do something he didn't want to do: speak up about his caregiving situation at work. That meant asking for more flexibility and time to get his parents settled. Unfortunately, the conversation with his boss did not go well. Phil's dedication and drive were questioned. He was told he might not be a "cultural fit." The boss refused to grant Phil's request for unpaid time off. Instead, he dou-bled down on Phil's year-end expectations. If he failed to deliver, his boss warned, Phil's job was on the line. Phil didn't want to have to choose between his job and caring for his parents. That just didn't seem fair. And it probably wasn't legal either.

Workplace Discrimination

Phil's boss not only dismissed Phil's reasonable request for support, he was possibly putting the company at risk too. Family responsibilities discrimination, or FRD, is one of the biggest challenges employers never see coming.[5] FRD refers to employment discrimination based on an employee's caregiving situation, such as pregnancy, caring for a child, or caring for a sick or disabled family member. These cases are on the rise, particularly eldercare discrimination, which has increased 650 percent in recent years.[6] A big part of the problem occurs when companies fail to implement policies and train front-line managers on how to support their caregiving employees. Not only do employers risk financial damage—employees in FRD cases were awarded close to half a billion dollars in verdicts over the last decade—but word travels fast.[7] Organizations that treat their caregiving employees poorly are not places most people want to work. Sooner or later, most of us will either be a caregiver or need care ourselves.

After Phil's discouraging meeting with his boss, he felt defeated but determined not to give up. Believing there must be something the company could do to help, he set up a meeting with human resources to explain his predicament. The HR director, a no-nonsense woman in her fifties, had a warm, knowing look that made you think she had seen it all. She listened to Phil's story with compassion and understanding. "Clearly," she said, "we need to do more training so that managers around here understand how to help employees in your situation." She said she would speak to Phil's boss to reeducate him about the company policies and resources for caregivers. Then the human resources director laid out the options.

First, she wondered if a change in schedule would allow Phil the time he needed to move his parents to Pittsburgh. Offering flexibility, or "flextime," is a crucial way for employers to help employees successfully juggle the demands of caregiving and work. When you're locked into a 9-5 workday without any wiggle room, you may end up among the statistics of caregivers who show up late to work—or not at all. As a caregiver, I managed to stay in the workforce all those years because of understanding bosses who allowed me the flexibility I needed to make it all work. Without that, the guilt on all fronts would have been overwhelming. But keeping your job and caring for your parent at the same time should not depend on being lucky enough to have an understanding manager. There's a reason the film *Horrible Bosses* touches a nerve. Most of us have been there, done that, and don't want to do it again.

So what are good employers doing to help people like Phil? They increasingly recognize that offering flexibility not only keeps their employees happy, but may also boost the bottom line. For every dollar invested in flextime, businesses can expect a return on their investment of between $1.70 and $4.34.[8] Still, there's plenty of fear out there that prevents people from speaking up. In 2014, support for flexibility in the workplace came from an unlikely source: the federal government. During the White House Summit on Working Families, President Barack Obama encouraged federal employers to expand flexible workplace policies, such as telecommuting and alternative work schedules. That meant federal employees would have the right to request flexibility without fear of retaliation. In fact, everyone *should* have that right. Keep in mind: you may not get exactly what you ask for, but you may get what you need to stay in the workforce.

Employer Response

During his sit-down with human resources, Phil learned about a range of benefits the company provided that his boss had never mentioned. Among them was backup dependent care for employees needing temporary in-home care for their children or adult family members anywhere in the country. And that included small rural towns like Shiner. The hourly rate was heavily subsidized by the company and included up to ten days of care per year. That might come in handy as Phil planned the next steps for his parents' move. The company also had an eldercare referral service, providing a list of nationwide options such as in-home care and senior housing. Good to know, since Phil would need help finding the right living arrangement for his parents when they relocated to Pittsburgh.

All of this came as a pleasant surprise after the less-than-helpful response from Phil's boss. Phil was grateful to know that his company was actually invested in keeping people like him employed and making their lives more manageable. But what Phil needed more than anything else was time. He needed time to figure out where to move his folks, work out the finances, and relocate them to Pittsburgh. Adjusting his hours just wouldn't cut it. Furthermore, Phil knew the job demanded his full-time attention, which he wasn't in a position to give right now. So Phil looked the human resources director in the eye and asked the question: "How can I take a break to care for my parents without losing my job?"

Family Leave

In 1993, the federal Family and Medical Leave Act (FMLA) was signed into law, ensuring eligible employees up to twelve weeks of unpaid leave per year. Reasons for eligibility include pregnancy, care of a newborn, and personal or family illness. Companies with fifty or more employees are now obligated by law to allow employees a protected leave of absence without pay.[9] But most people can't afford to go without pay for a few months while they care for a family member, even if they don't have to worry about losing their job. There are, however, a handful of states, including California, New Jersey, and Rhode Island, that have passed laws guaranteeing partially paid family leave through an employee-funded insurance program. While on leave, you'll collect only a portion of your salary, but it's definitely better than nothing.

Phil decided he would take advantage of the FMLA, which would give him the time he needed to resettle his parents. His job and the repairs on his house would just have to wait. Through his benefit at work, Phil got a list of senior housing options in the Pittsburgh area and started scoping them out. Eventually he found a continuing care retirement community nearby that would allow his parents to increase the level of care as their needs evolved. The sale of their home in Texas would help pay the entrance fee. While the move from Texas was emotional, Phil's parents made a surprisingly smooth adjustment to their new surroundings. His mother took advantage of the course offerings at the retirement community and signed up for a class on politics and ethics, which his father described as an oxymoron. Meanwhile, Phil's dad enrolled in a chair yoga class, which seemed to invigorate both his mind and body. Six weeks after the move, Phil's parents celebrated their sixty-fifth wedding anniversary with Phil by their side. "Not many couples reach this milestone," Phil said. "It was a gift to be with them. I felt so grateful that I found a way for them to age together with the care and the dignity they both deserve."

Solving the Work/Care Conflict

Phil's experience was not unique. He had a manager who was inflexible and dismissive of his requests. Phil's company had policies in place to support caregiving employees, but hadn't done a good job educating their managers about them, so what good did it do? Had Phil not received help through human resources, he probably would have had to choose between his job and caregiving, something many in the workforce are compelled to do. In fact, close to 40 percent of caregiving employees claim they work in inflexible environments and have been forced to reduce their work hours or quit.[10] That not only hurts employees, it costs employers as well. It is estimated that lost productivity, absenteeism, and workday interruptions due to caregiving cost U.S. businesses up to $33 billion annually. And that doesn't include the extra $13 billion per year in healthcare costs for caregiving employees, who get sick more often than their noncaregiving counterparts.[11] Sounds like a reason for employers to step up to the plate.

Employers are increasingly aware of the reality that caregivers come in many varieties. One employee may be rushing home to relieve the nanny while another may be calling Mom to make sure the home health aide arrived on time. All caregivers' needs matter. Until recently, those on the eldercare end of the age spectrum felt otherwise. Thankfully, times are changing. One reflection of this trend is an organization launched in 2010 called ReAct, which stands for Respecting a Caregiver's Time (www .respectcaregivers.org). ReAct is an employer-focused coalition dedicated to increasing awareness of the challenges faced by caregiving employees and establishing best practices in workplace eldercare. As a member of this organization, I have seen the tide slowly turn as employers accept their role in the family care equation. According to Drew Holzapfel, chairman of ReAct, "The work-care conflict is not an insurmountable problem. Employee caregivers can face rigid scheduling policies at work, stressful distractions at home, and see their own health decline from this demanding burden. With the right proactive policies and solutions, employers can drive a win-win."

Ask and You Might Receive

If you are among the many people like Phil, struggling to balance your job and caregiving, hopefully you're working for a good company. If not, it may be some small solace to know that you're not alone. So what can you do to make work *work*, at least a little better, and minimize the guilt and grief of feeling like you're failing on all fronts? The first step is to come out of the closet— because sooner or later you're going to be outed anyway. Talk to your manager and ask about workplace policies and benefits for caregiving employees. If your boss is not knowledgeable or responsive, go to human resources. If you work in a union shop, find out if the union is prioritizing family-friendly workplace benefits as part of its bargaining strategy. If you look hard enough, chances are you'll find a sympathetic ear somewhere in the organization to help you come up with a plan.

Like many caregivers, you may need to adjust your schedule, work remotely, or take time off. Maybe you'll learn about benefits that can really make a difference, like backup care, information and referral assistance, or in-home care management assessments. Some employers offer lunch-'n'-learn seminars and webinars so you can get some much-needed info and meet fellow caregivers in the process. Other organizations take it a step further and provide in-person consultations with senior care experts and caregiver support groups. So why don't you know about all this stuff? You may have received some emails or seen the information posted on your company's intranet. But you probably didn't pay attention or forgot about it, because until you are in the caregiving boat, you are not necessarily looking for a paddle.

Many larger organizations also have employee assistance programs (EAPs) that can be helpful, especially for stressed-out caregivers. EAPs provide a wide range of support for personal and work-related issues such as addictions, dependent care, legal needs, and emotional problems. It's confidential, so you don't have to worry about your boss or human resources knowing your business.

Sometimes, no matter what an employer claims to offer, it's just not a caregiver-friendly place to work. Maybe your boss is a jerk or your hours too set in stone. Ultimately, you must decide if it's possible to make work *work* while you're a caregiver. If it's not, maybe you need to consider a change and find a more flexible job or make some adjustments to your current one.

Paying attention to your own stress level is also important, and can help you avoid some potentially major missteps. A week after I took my father to work because the caregiver didn't show up, I had a sign from the universe that I was seriously overwhelmed. A particularly challenging client had been pushing my buttons for quite some time. Instead of setting appropriate limits, I was giving in to all her demands, at my own expense. After working extra hours trying to meet this client's expectations, I was dismayed to receive an email the next day with more complaints. I felt my blood pressure rise and needed to let off some steam. So I forwarded the client's email to a sympathetic colleague and wrote, "She's driving me up the *@&ing wall!" Only instead of "forward," I hit "reply."

After berating myself and profusely apologizing, I found this mortifying gaffe had some unintended positive consequences. It actually reset my relationship with the client in a much better direction. She felt bad that I was so frustrated and modified her approach. I also acknowledged that my current daily routine was not working. Going to the hospital to visit my mother at the end of a long workday, with Dad in tow, was just too much. So I adjusted my schedule, left work early, and cut myself some slack. And I learned another lesson the hard way— I've been really careful with email ever since.

We Are Each Other's Keeper

As caregivers in the workforce, the more we speak up and ask for support, the better off we all will be. But what if your employer is you and you can't afford to take time off? That was the case with Camille, a forty-year-old native of Haiti who had a job she loved that paid $12 an hour. Camille was a home health aide who believed caring for seniors was God's work. "I enjoyed hearing their stories and learning about their lives. I took the time to really listen and let them know their opinions matter," she said. "And I made them feel cared for and loved." While the pay was low and the demands high, Camille did not complain. Being a professional caregiver felt more like a calling than a job. But when her seventy-year-old mother was diagnosed with cancer, Camille felt unmoored. "My mom needed me and I needed to be with her." There was no backup care program or employer-supported eldercare to help Camille manage her work and her mother's care. "There was only me," Camille explained as she reflected on the fact that she had the right training for this unexpected role in life. Camille left her job and apartment and moved in with her mother, whom she cared for over the next three years, until her mother's death. Not long afterward, Camille returned to work for a company that offered benefits to their caregiving employees. "It's too late for me," laments Camille. "But I don't want others to go through what I did and leave a job they love because they have no choice."

Camille had a triple whammy. Compared to other demographic groups, low-income workers, minorities, and women are the most vulnerable to work/care conflicts. Because of their caregiving role, they are more likely to reduce their hours or leave the workforce altogether.[12] Working in restaurants, retail, factories, and healthcare, these workers are struggling to keep their heads above water and eke out a livable wage. When they become caregivers and their world turns upside down, like Camille's did, they may be out of luck. It's much harder to come forward and ask for support if you're at the bottom of the employment food chain.

Being your own best advocate may be a way to effect change and stay in the workforce, but it comes with a certain degree of risk. Not all workers feel empowered to ask for what they want, in the hopes of getting what they need. By speaking up and coming out of the shadows, we may also give voice to the voiceless caregivers out there. By looking out for ourselves, we are also looking out for each other. After all, we are all in this boat together.

EIGHT

The Art of Connection

Caring for a Loved One with Dementia

Too often we underestimate the power of a touch,
a smile, a kind word, a listening ear, an honest
compliment, or the smallest act of caring, all of which
have the potential to turn a life around.
—LEO BUSCAGLIA

We Won't Wait

In the fall of 2015, I had the opportunity to participate in an event sponsored by UsAgainstAlzheimer's, an organization dedicated to the relentless mission of finding a cure for Alzheimer's disease. The organization was founded by Trish and George Vradenburg, a wealthy, politically connected couple who decided to spend their personal fortune to achieve this audacious goal. Trish, whose mother died from the disease, was a former comedy sketch writer for television and didn't hesitate to in-fuse humor into the intensity of her passion. Referring to the fact that her children's inheritance is being funneled to this worthy cause, Trish explained, "Our daughter [who happened to be sitting in the audience] is just going to have to get used to rhinestones." Sadly, Trish died in 2017, but her crusade against Alzheimer's disease lives on. By lobbying government, industry, and the scientific community, the organization is sending a loud and clear message: *We won't wait. We* are all of us, members of the global community, both those already impacted by Alz-heimer's disease and dementia and those who recognize that we may be in the future. *We* are hoping to use our collective voice to encourage political leaders to fund re-search and treatment now so we can eradicate this terrible disease once and for all.

I was inspired by the event and met family caregivers and professionals in the field—most who'd been person-ally impacted by the disease and understood the toll it takes. The numbers alone are staggering: as of 2017, an estimated 5.5 million Americans have Alzheimer's disease, and 47 million people worldwide suffer from it. By 2050 these estimates are projected to triple and the direct cost to American society may exceed a trillion dollars—a price we all will pay in one way or another.[1] Although the disease does not discriminate, it disproportionately impacts women. Women are twice as likely to suffer from Alzheimer's and more than twice as likely to care for someone with the disease.[2] Despite these dire predictions, a nationally representative study indicated that dementia rates in the United States unexpectedly fell from 2000 to 2012. Even so, the greatest risk factor is age, and those over eighty-five are the most vulnerable. Without a cure, most of us fortunate enough to grow old will not be spared from this scourge. Over the course of a lifetime, we will likely care for someone with the disease or have it ourselves.

When my father first began showing signs of dementia, it was gradual, like a light rain before what would eventually become a monsoon. Initially we were not concerned about his forgetfulness, attributing it to his getting up in years. As many of my fellow boomers will attest, a certain amount of absent-mindedness is expected as we get older. We watch a Netflix film halfway through before we realize we've seen it before. Or we read a book, put it down for a few days, and then have to reread previous chapters to remember what the heck's going on. But dementia is different. It is a brain disease, not a manifestation of encroaching age. It robs victims of the ability to function as independent human beings, first gradually, then more rapidly as the monstrous malady runs its course.

When I describe the course of my father's illness, I typically use the term *dementia*, which includes a category of diseases characterized by a severe decline in mental functioning that interferes with daily life. We don't definitively know what type of dementia plagued my dad, but because of his history of hypertension and heart disease, we assume it may have been vascular dementia, the second most common variety. And perhaps my grandmother, who had a paranoid fixation that a gang was out to get her, suffered from Lewy body dementia, which has symptoms that include visual hallucinations and delusions. Back then it was just called senility. Alzheimer's is the most prevalent type of dementia, accounting for about 60 to 80 percent of all cases.[3] Today, through clinical examination and neuroimaging, a diagnosis can be made by a skilled memory disorder specialist with a high degree of accuracy. But once you have a diagnosis, there is no shying away from how grim this news is, because you are dealing with a progressive and ultimately fatal disease with no cure in sight.

In the early stages, short-term memory is among the first casualties. This can be particularly exasperating for caregivers, who find that they are listening to the same stories or responding to questions repeated over and over again. Information is not easily retained, which makes any kind of communication challenging. I recall my father's alarm when he woke up every morning to discover that my mother was in the hospital, where she'd been for a week, as if this was new and jarring news each day. Only when I made an actual sign, explaining the facts in a simple and straightforward manner, did my father gain some control over the situation, allowing his anxiety to eventually subside. As time progresses, the insidious disease will do more damage. Eating, bathing, walking, and going to the bathroom—activities of daily living that are so vital to identity and dignity—will become compromised. During the time my father lived with me, he could get dressed by himself with minimal help. He also was able to take his own shower, or so I thought, until one day I found water dripping from the dining room ceiling. When I went upstairs to check, I found my dad had forgotten to close the shower curtain. The bathroom floor was a lake. This incident, along with many to follow, signaled further decline and was a painful reminder of the relentless ferocity of his disease.

The Path to Connection

When words that once flowed fluidly are irretrievable or jumbled beyond comprehension, the path to connection becomes increasingly severed. During the middle stage of dementia, my father, a highly educated and articulate man, had difficulty following conversations and would often nod in feigned understanding when someone asked him a simple question. Eventually, communication becomes more elusive and the world increasingly out of reach for dementia's victims. In the last stage, many people, like my father, need constant care and oversight. They cannot communicate basic needs such as discomfort, hunger, or pain. They must rely on someone else to do what they can't do for themselves. They need a lifeline, no matter how small their world has become. We are that lifeline, because despite all that's been lost, the ability to love and be loved remains. If we are willing to open ourselves up to what Dr. Bill Thomas, a renowned geriatrician and healthcare innovator, refers to as "transcending the tragedy narrative and engaging with possibility," we may uncover what is still there.[4]

John Zeisel, PhD, in his book *I'm Still Here*, puts forth a radical new paradigm about understanding Alzheimer's and pushes us to reexamine our assumptions about the disease. The mind of someone with dementia, according to Zeisel, is a creative and active one.[5] Through stimulating the senses and engaging with the emotional self, caregivers can find a powerful path to connection. Creative outlets such as music and art can stimulate the brain and decrease agitation, isolation, and despair. Zeisel advocates a mix of nonpharmacological treatments along with standard medical care as the most effective approach to treat Alzheimer's and dementia. My dad tried a number of the available dementia medications, including Aricept and Namenda, which seemed to temporarily improve his short-term recall and alertness. But despite some mild improvements, no medication or treatment could change the steady, unalterable progression of the disease.

So we did what we could to keep my father as content as possible. Music always seemed to perk him up. During visits to the nursing home, my daughter would sing to my father and he would come alive. Through song, my daughter taught my father some Spanish (a language he did not speak)—remarkably, he would remember some of the words weeks later. Anyone who's watched Henry Dryer, an unlikely YouTube sensation from the film *Alive Inside*, may be awestruck by the power of music to awaken a ninety-year-old man with Alzheimer's who was largely cut off from the outside world. Henry—which also happens to be my father's name—had barely spoken a word in over ten years. When someone sets up an iPod program at his nursing home and Henry listens to Cab Calloway, the results are dramatic and inspiring. Henry somehow reacquires a lost part of his previous self through his connection to music. Music, according to Oliver Sacks, the famed neurologist and author, "can lift us out of depression or move us to tears. It is a remedy, a tonic, orange juice for the ear." Sacks went on to describe the impact music had on his neurologically impaired patients. "It can provide access, even when no medication can, to movement, to speech, to life."[6]

So does that mean that if you play your father's favorite song, you will get the same result? Maybe, maybe not. Finding a path to connection is different for everyone. In some instances, it will be truly amazing, like Henry's reaction to his favorite music, but more often it will be a subtle and fleeting awakening of mind and spirit. For the caregiver, it takes a certain amount of trial and error, patience, and hope. As family caregivers, we are so aware of all that's been lost that it's difficult to focus on what's still there. To adapt a glass is half full approach to dementia is no easy feat. But there is a difference between denial, not accepting the disease for what it is, and allowing ourselves the freedom to engage in ways beyond our normal mode of interaction. We must first accept that the person we love will not get better. We must make peace with this harsh reality before we can embrace and understand the altered version of the person we once knew. While the terrible scourge of dementia attacks both mind and memory—the very essence of a person's selfhood—there is still a part of identity that remains intact.

Even when language fails, we have the ability to connect and show our love in ways both genuine and profound. We can, according to Joanne Koenig Coste, an author and caregiving expert, "learn to speak Alzheimer's."[7] Coste defined the term *habilitation* as a framework for helping caregivers engage by focusing on remaining skills, simplifying the environment, and accepting our loved one's altered view of reality rather than imposing our own. In order to enter this world, as my mother did, we must first suspend our own hold on reality and learn a new way of communicating, even though it might involve some unusual things—like, perhaps, an imaginary companion.

My Father's Mistress

As physically debilitated as my father was, somehow he had become unfettered by the slavish devotion to reality to which the rest of us are confined. Instead, to while away the long, physically inactive hours in the nursing home, my father found a way to fill this void—with an imaginary mistress. Imagine my devoted mother's shock when she found out that a young, beautiful, and voluptuous paramour by the name of Cunégonde (pronounced kuh-nee-GOND-uh) had been entertaining my father with visits—regular visits, he said. And if you kept his mind engaged along this line of conversation, as my mother so diligently did, you'd find out they were conjugal visits!

Cunégonde, for those among us who have not read Voltaire, was the virtuous, innocent, beautiful, and servile woman idolized by Candide, the eponymous protagonist of Voltaire's novel. For my father, his imaginary companion Cunégonde acted in many dramatic roles. She was a playmate, lover, maternal figure, and most of all, as my dad himself explained, a source of solace. Also, the very mention of her would elicit my mother's warm and hearty laugh. My mother once asked my dad what he most appreciated about Cunégonde. "She has beautiful breasts," he quipped. "And she has a good disposition." Working with him to stay connected, my mother inquired, "Which is more important?" "You can't have one without the other!" blurted Dad. As they chortled together, it was comic proof that years of dementia had not dimmed the man's appreciation for the good things in life. Cunégonde, rather than threatening their relationship, was a source of comfort to them both. The mistress, friend, and caregiver provided my father with what my mother could not: ever-present companionship. My father's ability to combat the isolation of dementia by creating an imaginary mistress, who served as both salve and shield, expanded the confines of his constrained world and may have protected him from falling into despair.

Early on in the course of the disease, my father acknowledged the need to shift toward a different, more placid mode of existence. "I used to be type A, but now I'm not. I think senility suits me," my father said, to our astonishment. Although there was plenty of sadness and pain after the diagnosis, my father chose not to stay in that place. He was willing to let go of the burdens he had shouldered throughout his life and just be. My mother was able to provide a vital link to my father's history and connect the dots between his past and present, which he could not do on his own. She knew my father better than anyone and understood how the pain of his early years had shaped the man he had become.

My father was born in 1926 in Nuremberg, Germany, a city remembered as the site of infamous Nazi rallies and Hitler's subsequent rise to power. As a boy, my father recalled, he returned home one day along familiar streets, finding himself alone in a wildly cheering crowd and being commanded to raise his right arm to the shouts of "Sieg Heil!" as Adolf Hitler waved from an open window. It was only through the tenacity of my paternal grandmother, my Oma, that the family escaped the horrific fate that befell millions of Jews, including a number of my father's relatives, who lost their lives in the Holocaust. Upon arriving in New York City in 1938, my father struggled with feeling like an outsider and had to quickly assimilate into an exciting and unfamiliar world. His aptitude for learning soon became apparent and he was accepted into New York's City College, which he described as the "Harvard of the proletariat." After college, my father pursued a PhD in clinical psychology and subsequently devoted his professional life to working with mentally ill adults.

Though traumatized by his early experiences, my father had acquired skills of survival and adaptability that served him well throughout life and may have helped him cope with a debilitating disease. The "type A" person my father had once been was erased by dementia. In its place was an easygoing man who readily showed affection and would often greet my mother with a loving smile and a twinkle in his eye. This was an unforeseen gift that made it easier for my mother, my father's caregiver and lifeline, to carry on despite all the heartache. In this sense, we were lucky. But other dementia caregivers are not so fortunate; rather, they find they are caring for someone who is angry and contentious. Instead of appreciation, these caregivers are faced with constant criticism. How do you maintain your equanimity as a caregiver when instead of Dr. Jekyll, you are dealing with Mr. (or Mrs.) Hyde?

Anger Redirected

"Looking back," Hattie recalled, reflecting upon her mother's life, "my mom was not a good candidate for aging. The narcissistic injuries of growing old were tough for her to bear." Hattie's mother Faye had always cared a great deal about appearances. In high school, Faye was the pretty, popular cheerleader, the girl every guy wanted to take to the prom. After marrying her high school sweetheart, Faye had several children in quick succession, but motherhood was not a role that made her happy. "My mother was not a nurturing person. She was frequently critical and always seemed to be in competition with me and my sisters," Hattie explained. "And I for one never measured up."

Hattie had hoped to become an architect, but she did not pursue that path because her parents felt it was not an appropriate career for a woman. So instead, Hattie became a nurse. When Faye began showing signs of dementia, Hattie had medical skills and know-how, so much of the caregiving responsibilities fell on her shoulders rather than her siblings'. When Faye could no longer live on her own, Hattie moved her mother into an assisted living community. That worked okay for a while, but soon Hattie was getting calls during work about her mother's behavior. During "happy hour," Faye had gotten a little too happy and grabbed another resident's chardonnay. On another occasion, Faye had insulted an African American caregiver by lamenting that white people would soon become a minority. The most worrisome incident occurred when Faye pushed a resident during a brief altercation. "I was mortified," said Hattie. "And she was not any nicer to me. One time when I visited she called me a nit-faced jerk. That's the thanks I get for being a good daughter."

Hattie knew it was just a matter of time before her mother was going to get kicked out of the assisted living facility, so she began looking for a nursing home with a dementia unit, also known as special care units (SCUs). Some assisted living communities have memory care units that can handle late-stage dementia, whereas others are equipped to care only for people in the early stages of the disease. Since 60 percent of nursing home residents have Alzheimer's disease or dementia, the demand for specialized care is on the rise.[8] A number of states have enacted legislation requiring oversight of SCUs, ensuring that quality standards are in place and professionals have received proper training in dementia care. When my father was in a nursing home, residents with dementia were placed in the same unit, but the care was not specifically designed to meet their needs. If you are dealing with behaviors like the kind Faye was exhibiting, a specialized care unit can make a big difference. For example, shortly after Faye arrived at the facility, she became agitated and insisted she had to go on a trip. Rather than talk her out of it, the aide brought Faye a suitcase and helped her pack. The aide asked Faye where she was going and what she planned to do once she got there. Later, when Hattie arrived for a visit, she was stunned to see her contented mother with a fully packed suitcase by her side. When Hattie learned about the aide's approach and how it quickly calmed her mother down, she felt reassured she had chosen the right place.

During the year that Faye spent at the nursing home, her angry outbursts did not disappear, but they significantly subsided. The staff at the nursing home viewed problematic behavior as an expression of an unmet need and felt it was their job to figure out what was going on and what to do about it. Faye still gave the staff a hard time on occasion, but they tried not to struggle with her. Instead, when Faye became angry, the staff redirected her with activities that had a calming effect, such as listening to classical music or playing bingo. Hattie learned a lot from the nursing home team's approach and sought out information and resources so she could communicate better with her mother. She read *The 36-Hour Day*, a comprehensive guide for families caring for people with

Alzheimer's disease and dog-eared the sections on combativeness and caregiving.[9] She contacted the Alzheimer's Association hotline and spoke with a helpful staff person who suggested caregiving strategies and directed Hattie to a support group. She learned not to meet anger with anger and was able to maintain a positive connection with her mother by speaking in a calm and soothing voice using slow, short sentences. As the disease progressed, Hattie relied more on wordless communication, discovering that maintaining eye contact while gently touching her mother's hand brought a smile to her face. Hattie also found that giving her mother a sense of control, even when it meant offering small choices, was a good way of avoiding conflict. Should we visit in the courtyard or the day room? Would you like to listen to Vivaldi or Chopin? Do you want to wear the blue sweater or the brown one?

In time, Hattie was able to dislodge herself from the mother/daughter cycle of anger and hurt that had characterized their relationship for so many years. "In the end, I know she appreciated I was there for her," said Hattie. Several months after Faye died, Hattie had a dream that a woman was walking toward her. As the woman came closer, Hattie could see she had a huge smile on her face and realized it was her mother. "I had made peace with her," Hattie reflected. "I was a dutiful daughter. I cared for my mother and I feel good about that. It took a lot of energy but I don't have any regrets."

As a nurse, Hattie was not unprepared for the possibility that her mother might succumb to some form of dementia as she aged. She'd seen it before: the early memory loss and slow steady progression of a disease with a growing number of victims. She knew that growing old was risky business. If you live long enough, something's going to get you. But who would imagine a forty-something-year-old coming down with Alzheimer's disease? Daisy Duarte (who gave me permission to use her real name) certainly didn't. After a devastating diagnosis, however, Daisy's worst fears would soon become her day-to-day reality.

Daisy's Story

When Daisy's mother first became forgetful, the doctors thought she might be depressed. Daisy's mother Sonia was in her late forties and was a beloved teacher's aide in the Chicago school system. Daisy didn't think her mother was depressed, but she knew something wasn't right. "We would be driving to church and my mother thought she left the coffee pot on or the door unlocked. No matter how late we were, we had to turn back." Other worrisome changes followed. Sonia loved to cook big pots of rice and fried chicken to bring to church, but now she had forgotten the recipe. When Sonia's speech lapsed into gibberish and her moods became volatile, Daisy needed answers. So she took her mother to a memory disorder clinic for a thorough evaluation. The results were shocking. Sonia was diagnosed with early-onset Alzheimer's—a less common and more virulent form of the disease. Early onset affects an estimated two hundred thousand people in the United States—about 5 percent of Americans who have Alzheimer's disease. Also known as familial Alzheimer's disease, early onset is often linked to a genetic hereditary mutation.[10] Like many in the Latino community, where the disease is still cloaked in shame, Daisy did not know much about Alzheimer's before her mother's diagnosis. But as she discovered more, it all started making sense. A number of Daisy's relatives on her mother's side had died from the disease, all at relatively young ages.

Daisy decided to quit her job running a sports bar to become a full-time caregiver. "My mother did not want to leave Chicago but eventually agreed to move in with me and my partner in Springfield, Missouri. She was initially critical of my lifestyle," Daisy explained. "But my partner was a huge support and helped me care for my mom." In time, Sonia came to love Daisy's partner too. "My partner and I would tuck my mother into bed every night and say *Te amo*—I love you." Daisy credits her faith in God for helping her cope with all the stresses of being a full-time caregiver. In addition to the physical and emotional challenges, Daisy was in a hole financially. Sonia's modest pension barely covered food and rent, and Daisy still had to pay for medications, diapers, wipes, and basic house-hold expenses.

But the biggest source of stress was yet to come. Daisy made a brave and terrifying decision to get tested for the disease herself. The news was devastating. Daisy learned she had the same genetic mutation as her mother. That meant that by the time Daisy was sixty-five, she would have Alzheimer's disease. How do you go on after learn-ing such a fate awaits you? Some days, Daisy acknowl-edges, she feels filled with despair. "I see how people go the exit route," she says. But through her faith in God and the support of a loving partner, Daisy found the strength to choose another path. As an Alzheimer's ad-vocate and activist, Daisy champions the needs of family caregivers and raises awareness in the Latino community. She works with the organization UsAgainstAlzheimer's to advocate for increased funding for Alzheimer's treatment and research. And she cherishes the fact that she is taking good care of her mother and probably prolonging her life. "She is not my first mom. I accept that person is gone. But she is my second mom. And I love her just as much. Every day, I am grateful that I still have her with me."

The Healing Power of Connection

In May 2016, I attended an event focused on dementia that actually lifted my spirits. It was called Disrupt Dementia, part of a national tour by Dr. Bill Thomas, founder of the Eden Alternative, an innovative approach to de-institutionalize and humanize long-term care. Thomas and his team of activists, actors, musicians, and poets barnstormed the country celebrating aging in an attempt to transform the way we think about dementia. Thomas espouses the Hippocratic maxim that you should know the person with the disease, not just the disease itself. Thomas shifts away from the notion of caregiver and sufferer—recognizing that a person with dementia is still capable of giving and receiving love. Through creativity, community, and emotional connections, people with dementia can combat isolation and remain engaged. When it comes to dementia patients, Thomas believes, "connection is their safety."

My mother understood this crucial need for connection: her relationship with my father survived and even thrived during the course of his illness. She could accept my dad as he was and did not try to remake him into the man he once had been. She rarely corrected him and did not require that he be steeped in reality. This allowed them the freedom to journey together—at least through the lens of my father's imagination. Remarkably, my father achieved a sort of Zen in the final years of his dementia. On his birthday the year before he died, I asked my father how it felt to turn eighty-five. "Good," he replied cheerfully. "I love food. I love life. And my mind is still working." This from a man who lived in a nursing home, confined to a wheelchair, eating ground-up food for breakfast, lunch, and dinner. In his own way, my father was a disrupter of dementia, helped along by an imaginary and ever-present mistress and a real-life caregiver who served as his loving and devoted lifeline to the world.

NINE

Caring for the Parent Who Couldn't Care for You

All I want is what everybody else wants.
You know, to be loved.
—RITA HAYWORTH

Not long ago, my friend Morgan's father died after a long bout with Parkinson's disease. Morgan rarely spoke about her father, who had abandoned the family; his existence seemed shrouded in mystery. She often praised her mother, who was left to raise four children on her own. The little I knew of Morgan's father was that he was abusive, selfish, a tyrant at times. He had left when Morgan was just five years old, so her memories of him, while painful, were dim. It was more than fifty years before Morgan saw her father again, during the last year of his life. It was far from a Hollywood reunion, and the sadness and anger had not disappeared. But a frail old man dependent on caregivers for his day-to-day needs had replaced the strong, ferocious patriarch of Morgan's early childhood. Morgan never tried to undo the hurt and pain. Nor did she take on the role of primary caregiver. Instead, she tried to learn what she could of this man—a father in name only, but the only father she'd ever known. While it felt strange, Morgan managed to connect with this wrecking ball of a human, who had never so much as kissed her goodnight.

Morgan's experience was so vastly different from my own. My father, who could be emotionally volatile at times, was nonetheless an attentive, loving parent devoted to his wife and children. Dementia brought out my father's sweet nature, which made the burdens of caregiving easier to bear. After hearing Morgan's story, I wondered what it would be like to care for a parent who had not cared for you. Morgan's father had deliberately and inexplicably severed the most powerful and lasting of human bonds—the connection between parent and child. How can you ever reconcile that choice and find it possible to forgive your parent? What if your parent had acted not out of intent or malice but from a place of addiction, mental illness, or both? If you suffered through a childhood of neglect or abuse—whatever the reason—could you ever be able to care for your tormentor? Are you responsible to care for your parent at all? And how do you handle all the anger and resentment and choose a path that doesn't put your sanity and health at risk?

A number of family caregivers I interviewed for this book had a history of troubled relationships with a parent. Some grew up with an abusive, alcoholic parent and were faced with a difficult decision when their mother or father needed care. Others were struggling to care for a parent with mental illness, often undiagnosed, whose incapacities only worsened with age. Assuming the care of a parent who didn't adequately parent you is a complex and highly personal decision. There are risks: adults who endured childhood mistreatment are more vulnerable to depression when caring for their abusive parent.[1] Even so, most folks feel it is their responsibility to assume the caregiving role, and they rarely call it quits. In these delicate and difficult scenarios, there's no clear right or wrong. But there's often plenty of anguish mixed in with a big dose of guilt.

Following Your Own Footsteps

Karen, a successful businesswoman, grew up in an Irish Catholic family that was "swimming in guilt." Her father, whom she described as a "life-long alcoholic" and a "charmer," had molested Karen as a child. Karen recalls that she and her siblings were all abused in one way or another while their mother looked the other way, desperately pretending that everything was okay. "There was a lot of anger and resentment growing up but nothing got discussed openly," said Karen. She describes a horrible relationship with both her parents, who often made her feel unloved and worthless. "My mother used to tell me I was a mistake, and I believed her," she said. As an adolescent, Karen found numerous ways to rebel, such as wearing hippie-style clothes and no bra. This enraged her mother, who wanted Karen to dress "like a preppy." In young adulthood, Karen became increasingly self-destructive and eventually became addicted to alcohol and drugs. The guilt and shame that were so central to Karen's identity made her feel trapped and condemned to repeat the dysfunction of her past.

"I was following in my father's footsteps," reflects Karen, who has been in recovery for over twenty years. The disease of addiction is complex, resulting from both genetic and environmental factors, both of which affected Karen. And the combined triggers of trauma, chronic stress, and repeated exposure are a triple threat.[2] To survive, Karen needed to find a way to live her life—a way different from the one she knew. Through the twelve-step fellowship of Alcoholics Anonymous, Karen found a path toward health and healing. Years later, the lessons from recovery came in handy when Karen's aging parents were both afflicted with chronic illnesses. For Karen, assuming the role of caregiver was a risk, but perhaps also an opportunity. Karen knew she had to compartmentalize her past and avoid being triggered into relapse. She had to focus on the present and figure out how to help her parents without hurting herself. She knew she could not undo the damage that had already been done. But she was no longer a victim either. And that felt empowering.

Several years after Karen and her siblings left home, their parents separated but never divorced, because, according to Karen, "they were too Catholic." As bad as the marriage was, her parents had been each other's sole source of support. Now alone, both her parents were declining. Karen's father had been diagnosed with a form of dementia considered irreversible, brought on by years of alcohol abuse. Karen encouraged her father to seek treatment for his addiction. She shared her own path toward recovery and identified treatment centers that specialized in older adults. Karen knew that her father's struggle was far from unique. Approximately 17 percent of older adults misuse alcohol and prescription drugs: it is one of the fastest-growing and least recognized health problems in this country.[3] According to Dr. Harry Haroutunian, author of *Not as Prescribed: Recognizing and Facing Alcohol and Drug Misuse in Older Adults*, family members often dismiss their parents' addicted behavior by reasoning they'll never change. Or they think their parents will die soon anyway and might as well enjoy themselves while they still can. But Karen knew her father's drinking was not a form of enjoyment. It was a disease. And it was steadily poisoning him to death.

Despite her efforts and good intentions, Karen could not save her father from himself. She and her siblings eventually moved their father into an assisted living community with a memory disorder unit, where he could receive the care he needed. "He was always scheming to get alcohol, and once in a while he succeeded. He never slowed down his antics," she said. "Once I got a call that he'd jumped into bed with one of the female residents." Karen struggled to be a good daughter but was often overcome with guilt and sadness. Her visits to her father were sporadic. Sometimes she would arrive at the assisted living facility and cry for an hour in the parking lot before she could bring herself to go in. Other times, she would turn around and go home, then send flowers instead. The feelings were as inexplicable as they were real: "Somehow, there was a part of me that still loved him, despite all that he had done."

Caregiving, more than almost any other role in our lives, takes us back to our roots and to the roles we played within our families of origin, explains Eleanor Cade, author of *Taking Care of Parents Who Didn't Take Care of You*.[4] Our family dynamics may seem fixed in time, threatening to suck us back to a period when chaos and dysfunction were all that we knew. For Karen, stepping into the role of parental caregiver triggered feelings of helplessness and shame that stemmed from a history of neglect and abuse. But she was no longer that same vulnerable child, powerless to alter her circumstances. She had a network of support: a trusted sponsor from AA and a therapist who helped her navigate the messy emotional terrain of caring for a destructive parent. For a while, Karen thought things were going okay. She was managing her father's care and her own complicated emotions about caring for him.

Then the other shoe dropped. Karen's mother, only sixty-two at the time, suffered a stroke. At first, things went from bad to worse. The stroke caused aphasia, which impaired her mother's ability to communicate. Frustrated, Karen's mother did not initially cooperate with treatment, which further decreased her mobility. But after three months in a rehab facility, the course of events unexpectedly changed. "It was like a lightning bolt hit my mother's brain," Karen explained. "Instead of my mother's bitterness, she began showing a kindness I had never experienced from her before. In response, I was able to find a well of compassion I didn't know was possible."

Karen's caregiving experience did not heal old wounds, but it did help her gain perspective and focus more on the present. After her parents died, Karen grieved for the family she had always wanted but never had. "I had to come to terms with my parents' profound limitations. I did not think I could ever forgive them," Karen said. "But the recovery process demanded I try." Seeing her parents as vulnerable and dependent on her for care lessened the anger she had harbored for so many years. Toward the end of her parents' lives, Karen learned more about their histories—her father's traumatic experience in the Korean War and her mother's hardscrabble upbringing in the Depression Rust Belt. Knowing more about her parents' past did not excuse what they had done, but it shed light on who they were and the hardships they had endured. "My relationship with my parents was never going to be based on honesty and trust," Karen acknowledged. "But I came to accept my mother and father and I was no longer fighting with them—or myself. I had achieved some degree of acceptance and peace. I guess I'll settle for that."

When it comes to caregiving, too much focus on past wrongs can rob the present of any redeeming opportunities, says Dr. Mark Agronin, geriatric psychiatrist and author.[5] Over the course of a lifetime, our connection to our parents requires reinvention so that we don't remain stuck in childhood perceptions. This relational shift is particularly important for caregivers who choose to care for parents who did not adequately care for them. But not everyone can make this transition. Sometimes the risks of caring for a neglectful or abusive parent are just too great. When a parent is so toxic, the proximity of caregiving may threaten to cause grave psychological harm. In those situations, the caregiver may feel that the only real choice, as drastic as it seems, is to walk away.

Opting Out: A Tough Choice

"I was an incredibly difficult kid. Those are just the facts," explains Dylan, a shy twenty-eight-year-old who works as a software tester for a tech start-up. "My mother's alcoholism started around the time I was born. And the stress of raising me certainly didn't help much. Growing up, my problems sounded like alphabet soup—ADD, ADHD, LD [learning disabilities], all mixed in with anxiety and depression," Dylan recalls. "For a long time, I thought I was the cause of my mother's problems."

Dylan never knew from day to day which mother he would find. Some days his mother seemed cheery, even though her speech was slurred and her thoughts incoherent. Other days she would be angry, screaming at Dylan for the slightest infraction, such as leaving Legos strewn across the floor or forgetting to switch off the light in the bathroom. But the most disturbing version of his mother was the one who crashed on the couch, oblivious to Dylan's needs or his very existence. "I kept upping the ante to get her attention," Dylan recalls. "One time I threw a toy across the room so hard that it broke the window. She woke up, yelled at me, and then went to her bedroom to sleep in peace." Dylan describes his father, on the other hand, as the "master of denial." When his mother developed tremors related to her alcohol abuse, Dylan's father said it was Parkinson's disease. The denial was pervasive; signs of worsening disease, such as falls and blackouts, were always explained away.

Congressman Patrick Kennedy, who grew up in a family plagued with addiction, knows the power of denial all too well. In his book *A Common Struggle*, Kennedy says that people often talk about "denial" as if it's a passive thing, a path of least resistance. "Denial is actually really aggressive. It's hard work," Kennedy notes.[6] Dylan remembers the time when his family's denial finally stopped working. His mother was hospitalized after a fall and the extent of her disease became evident. Multiple trips to rehab and AA meetings achieved only short-lived sobriety.

When Dylan was in his early twenties, trying to figure out what to do with his life, his family, tenuously held together for so long, began to fall apart. His older sister moved out of state and broke off ties with their mother. Dylan's father, after twenty-five years of marriage, filed for divorce. That left Dylan alone to assume the role of his mother's caretaker, at a time when he was barely able to care for himself. "I should have left home when my father moved out," Dylan reflects. "I wanted so bad to help my mother but I didn't know how." Dylan did what he could. He hid the alcohol and took his mother to the hospital when things got really bad. Despite all the tension, there were some good times too. "We both loved the cat and would laugh at his crazy stunts. We could go out for dinner and enjoy each other's company," Dylan recalls. But there were many dark moments and frequent fights. After a while, the battles took a menacing turn. On one occasion, Dylan threatened to throw a chair at his mother if she didn't stop screaming. When she continued to yell, he pushed her. Although his mother wasn't seriously injured, it was a terrifying incident: Dylan was shocked by the extent of the anger he had been harboring for so long. Overcome with guilt, he realized he could no longer safely care for his mother. He needed to take some time to sort out his own life. To do so, Dylan chose to cut off contact with his mother. What he didn't know was just how little time she had left.

Determined to escape from the dark emotional place he'd inhabited, Dylan sought therapy and started to exercise. He attended Al-Anon, a support organization for family and friends of alcoholics. Although he kept a distance, he stayed in touch with his mother's close circle of friends, who continued to support and care for her. Meanwhile, his mother's condition deteriorated, and she was hospitalized with severe kidney damage. When Dylan heard the news, he knew he had to see her again. During the visit, which turned out to be their last, Dylan's mother told him he was a good person. "She took responsibility for her life and didn't want me to blame myself. I did, of course. But after she died, I worked on forgiving myself and trying to forgive her."

Dylan wishes he could have been more available to his mother during the last months of her life. He wishes he had the opportunity to explain why he acted the way he did. "I always imagined that one day in the future we would talk." But looking back, Dylan does not think he could have done anything differently. He cared for his mother as best he could and, at some point, he needed to save himself. The regrets involved in that choice, he says, will stay with him for the rest of his life.

Dylan is among the 25 percent of family caregivers who are part of the millennial generation, born between 1982 and 2004. He describes himself as "mature in odd ways" and claims that not much gets to him since nothing is worse than what he went through. Therapy has helped him put his life experience in perspective and avoid being driven by his emotions. But the scars of growing up with an alcoholic parent are still raw. Dylan has not completely forgiven his mother, who died at the age of sixty-four from complications related to alcoholism. It took years for Dylan to realize that the disease of addiction had robbed him of his mother. In her place was a lost woman who was not capable of caring for him, because she was too busy destroying herself.

Those, like Dylan, raised by an impaired or neglectful parent are at risk of being embittered by the trauma they endured. Making peace with your parent does not require forgiving their sins. Seeing your parent as a highly flawed mortal rather than a monster may help. Over time, Dylan grew more curious about his mother's life. He learned that she grew up with an alcoholic father who denigrated and devalued her throughout childhood and beyond. She had embraced motherhood, wanting to provide her children with what she herself had never had. Sadly, Dylan's mother was unable to escape her own demons and fell victim to the same terrible disease that claimed her father.

As an adult, Dylan understood that his mother was not a bad person even though she did bad things. The conflicting emotions he felt toward her were just going to have to live inside him—side by side. They could not be ignored or reasoned away. At his mother's funeral, Dylan talked about their relationship and did not censor his feelings. He drew gasps from the mourners as he spoke with raw honesty: "I never hated anyone so much in my entire life. And I never loved anyone so much either."

As Dylan's eulogy so dramatically illustrates, relationships are rarely all good or all bad. According to Dr. Richard A. Friedman, professor of clinical psychiatry at Weill Cornell Medical College, "Even the most abusive parents can sometimes be loving, which is why severing a bond should be a tough, and rare, decision."[7] Given that 80 percent of long-term care in this country is provided by unpaid family members, caring for our parents, even the difficult ones, remains a cultural expectation. And in some states it may even be the law. There are twenty-eight states that currently have "filial support or responsibility" laws that require adult children to provide financial support for their parents if the parents are unable to pay for care. Although these laws are rarely enforced, there are cases in which adult children have been required to pay unpaid nursing home bills or other debts.

The law recognizes that if a parent abused or neglected a child, there is no reciprocal duty for the adult children to support the parent.[8] But what can they do? In the most extreme cases, adult children may request to have court-ordered conservators or guardians appointed to assume responsibility for a parent's financial and health-related decisions. This is usually a last resort and most people, especially those dutiful daughters, do what they can even if they don't get much back in return.

The Emotional Roller Coaster

Growing up, Carla knew there was something wrong with her mother. Uneventful days were a gift, but as time went on there were fewer of those. Her mother's wrath, like a tidal wave crashing to shore, would destroy any semblance of normalcy Carla clung to. When that happened, Carla and her younger sister would play hide-and-seek, hoping their mother would not find them. But she always did.

Carla recalls that when her mother was depressed it wasn't as bad. She would lie in bed all day, passive and seemingly harmless, like a rag doll. But the other end of the emotional roller coaster was often terrifying. Her mother would become giddy and then fly into a rage, taking Carla and her sister hostage. Meanwhile, Carla's father was kind but avoidant, "like an ostrich with his head in the sand." He stayed clear of the tsunami when it struck, unable to protect Carla and her sister from the brunt of their mother's mental illness, which went undiagnosed and untreated for years.

Carla's mother was eventually diagnosed with bipolar disorder, a chronic condition characterized by periods of depression followed by elevated and volatile moods. As adults, Carla and her sister tried to persuade their mother to seek treatment and take medication. Instead, she took nutritional supplements that, Carla joked, "gave her very expensive pee." Carla tried desperately to get her mother to accept help, but those efforts were typically thwarted. "My mother fired so many doctors. We were always starting over at zero." And her mother took her frustration out on Carla, whom she sometimes blamed for all her problems. These hurtful attacks took a toll. Soon, Carla found herself snapping at her husband and kids. One day, Carla's twelve-year-old daughter accused Carla of being just like

Grandma—a stunning slap in the face. Carla apologized and at the same time vowed to make a change. She gave her mother an ultimatum: "I won't see you until you follow through with treatment and get the help you need." With great difficulty, Carla stuck to her guns. A year went by before she would see her mother again.

There are approximately 8.4 million Americans, like Carla, who provide care to an adult family member with emotional or mental health issues. Close to two-thirds of these folks report a high level of emotional stress.[9] If you are one of the 8.4 million, you've got a tough road ahead. First, you are more likely to feel isolated and overburdened by the sheer demands and complexity of this type of care. The stigma of mental illness may make it harder for you to seek out much-needed help and support. Finding quality mental health care is no easy feat, and getting it covered by insurance may be a battle in itself. Even when a diagnosis is made and appropriate treatment found, your parent, like Carla's mother, may simply opt out. Compound all these obstacles with an angry or abusive parent and you may be putting your own mental health at risk. When that happens, where do you turn?

During the year that Carla cut off contact with her mother, she did something important for herself. She got into therapy. She needed to sort out the guilt from her agonizing decision to take a break. She wondered whether her pervasive feelings of insecurity and self-doubt were directly related to growing up with an erratic, emotionally imbalanced mother. Through psychotherapy, Carla became aware of the anger and sadness she had been living with for so long. "There was so much I needed as a child that I didn't get," Carla reflected. "Stability and predictability are so important for children and I try so hard to provide that for my kids." But Carla also understood that where you come from does not have to determine who you are and where you are going. She sought out ways to achieve equanimity in her life, despite the effects of a stormy upbringing. She started to meditate and pay attention to the way her body reacted to stress. She took an eight-week course called Family-to-Family, offered through the National Alliance on Mental Illness (NAMI), that taught strategies and coping skills for people caring for mentally ill family members.

Meanwhile, Carla kept in touch with her father, who continued to take care of her mother. There seemed to be no limits to her father's capacity to give, which both frustrated and amazed Carla. Her father's excessive caregiving may have kept her mother alive, but it also may have enabled her to resist help and remain ill. All the same, Carla was deeply moved by her father's unflinching and unconditional devotion. "We should all be so lucky to be that loved," she thought.

Later, when Carla's mother was admitted to a psychiatric hospital following a severe manic episode, Carla decided it was time to see her again. It had been a year, and Carla felt better equipped to handle the abuse that was sure to come. Instead, her mother's eyes welled with tears when Carla reappeared after so long. Carla could see that her mother's steely resistance had eroded. The health crisis had, quite unexpectedly, created an opening, and her mother was finally willing to acknowledge her illness and accept help. That help came in the form of a competent and compassionate psychiatrist who referred to the disease of bipolar disorder as "a wild horse to ride." The doctor explained that untreated, the horse was a bucking bronco. But if Carla's mother was willing to wear a saddle—which in this case meant medication and therapy —she'd still be in for a ride, but she'd be able to hold the reins.

With the support of a good psychiatrist, Carla's mother got into treatment for her illness. This eased the conflict between mother and daughter and led to a less combustible relationship. While her mother's rough edges had softened, they had not fully disappeared, and Carla was determined to protect herself from further assault. That meant maintaining a protective distance and resisting the inclination to be a savior. The year of separation from her mother had helped Carla recognize what she could change and accept what she could not. She could not heal her mother's pain or fill her heart with love. The unkindness Carla had experienced would never go away, but it did not have to define her either. For the remaining years of her mother's life, Carla took care of her as best she could. "I did it more for myself than for her. I didn't want any regrets once she died."

In the end, Carla was proud of the way she handled herself. There were some silver linings; she gave her children what she herself had not had—a stable and loving mother. She formed a closer bond with her sister, who had also suffered from their mother's abuse. She gained a grudging admiration for her father while feeling sad for him at the same time. "He made the choice to stick it out. I think he really loved my mom. But to stay with her, he had to put up with a lot of crap. That was his choice to make. As for me, my putting up with crap days are over."

A Path toward Healing

Caring for a parent who did not care for you may feel like your last chance for connection, no matter how imperfect that connection may be. Repairing the damage and fixing what's broken is rarely achievable. Caring for your uncaring parent as best you can might provide you with some comfort and free you from the cycle of anger and hurt that can threaten your soul. At the same time, you must protect yourself. Caregivers who experienced maltreatment at the hands of an abusive parent are particularly vulnerable to depression when they step into the caregiving role. While the Ten Commandments call on us to honor our father and mother, we must also honor ourselves. Everything in your life is interconnected, and putting yourself in harm's way may harm you as well as those around you. As fellow caregivers, we can hardly judge those like Dylan who make the decision to walk away. You have to recognize when you are at your limit. Reaching out for help and support can make a difference. Finding a good therapist, hiring caregivers to pitch in, and joining a support group can help you manage the stress and demands of caring for a parent who didn't adequately care for you.

None of us gets to choose the parents we are given in this world. Your "Mommy Dearest," like the allegedly abusive Joan Crawford, may be far from the loving mother you feel you deserved. You can't change your parents, and in most cases, you can't rescue them either. But you can rescue yourself from a cycle of pain and hurt that threatens to define your life. You can focus on the present and choose not to be broken by the past. You may even find some kernels of good, despite all that was bad. The process of aging, illness, and decline may alter a parent's character or self-understanding—occasionally in a beneficial way—opening the door to connections that can even become gratifying. In any case, whatever your path toward healing, it is possible to find compassion for your very flawed parent—and for yourself.

TEN

How to Care for Ourselves Too

When the well's dry, we know the worth of water.
—BENJAMIN FRANKLIN

Several years ago I was conducting a seminar entitled "Caring for the Caregiver." I went through the usual spiel, explaining how to put yourself on the "to do" list and pay attention to your own needs. I showed a slide with a picture of a flight attendant instructing passengers to put on their own oxygen mask before attempting to assist another person. Makes sense, right? If you're running out of air, how are you going to save anyone else? Then I glanced at the faces of the audience and saw blank stares. Some folks were even looking at their phones. Here I was trying to demonstrate one of the most important themes in caregiving—learning to care for you—and no one was paying attention.

Instructing people to care for themselves can often fall on deaf ears and may even feel like an added burden to already overworked caregivers. All that treacly advice about "me time" sounds good in theory, but it's tough to put into practice. As I observed the audience disengage, I knew I had to bring the issue of self-care to life and stop spouting platitudes. So I decided to share my personal story. Years earlier, when I was caring for my dad, I was overwhelmed and quick to put my own needs on the back burner. As Friedrich Nietzsche famously said, "That which does not kill us, makes us stronger." I thought soldiering on through a daily dose of demands and mustdos was the only path forward. But that approach did not make me stronger. In fact, it made things worse.

When Your Body Says, "Listen Up"

Since the age of sixteen, I've suffered from chronic daily headaches, which fluctuate from mildly annoying to downright disabling. I have seen numerous specialists, including neurologists, physical therapists, chiropractors, and acupuncturists—along with a shrink or two. I have tried countless medications, exercise, and diet regimens, even

Botox injections in my scalp and neck. Some treatments provided short-term relief, but nothing stops the daily throb that is my constant companion. I have lived by the motto that just because you have a pain doesn't mean you need to be a pain. As a result, most people in my life have no idea that I have headaches. For the most part, I keep it to myself.

One day when I was seeing my neurologist for a regularly scheduled appointment, my doctor deviated from his usual laconic manner and asked me a few questions about my life. I explained that like many forty-somethings, my plate was full. I worked full-time, had three kids, and helped care for my dad, who was living with me while my mother recuperated from hip surgery. "Hmmmm," the doctor muttered disapprovingly. "That's too much." "Excuse me?" I said defensively. "That's my life. No different from a lot of other women out there." "That may be," the doctor replied. "But your body is telling you something. Your headaches are getting worse and the medications aren't helping much. It might be time to slow down a bit." Annoyed, I pegged him as the guy who just doesn't get it. But in time, his message sank in.

When I went back for my next appointment, the headaches had increased in frequency and intensity. I asked the doctor if he had any suggestions for alleviating the pain, besides taking more pills. "Have you tried meditating?" he asked. "Oh, brother," I thought. "He must be grasping for straws if he thinks going to an imaginary happy place will make one whit of difference." But I had nothing to lose. "No, but I'm willing to give it a try," I said, feeling more resigned than optimistic. Over the next three months I regularly visited a psychologist trained in the art and science of meditation and biofeedback. I meditated twice a day for twenty minutes at home and at work. I learned to pay attention to my breathing as a way of quieting my overstuffed mind. I learned to be comfortable with stillness instead of racing through my day, hurtling from one task to another. And I gave myself permission to stop *doing*, at least for a brief period twice a day, and focus on *being*. Did my headaches disappear as a result? No, and neither did the stress of being a working caregiver. But it did help. The meditation made me calmer and may have lessened the headache pain too. The brief reprieve from the tyranny of tasks felt healing. Like many caregivers, I had been piling onto my overloaded plate without considering the cost.

Advice You Can't Ignore

As caregivers, we may ignore advice to take care of ourselves, but we do so at our own peril. We each have to replenish our reserves of strength and compassion or else our well will run dry. Caregiver stress is real. It can result in illness, addiction, depression, and social isolation. According to the American Psychological Association, caregivers report significantly higher levels of stress than the general population and perceive themselves to be in poor health.[1] They are more vulnerable to chronic health problems and physical injury. And they are less likely to sign up for a Pilates class at the gym, which they have no time to join. They are less inclined to seek preventive health measures *at exactly the age when those measures can be life-saving.*

It's easy to run yourself ragged when you are a caregiver. It happens when you don't consciously protect yourself from all the risks. The tightness in your chest, the frequent spats with your spouse, and the Ambien you pop to sleep through the night may be signs that something is amiss. When did you last say no to something you needed to do so you could say yes to something you wanted to do? It's not easy when you are *the one.* The one to take your mother to the doctor, get the kids to soccer practice, shop, cook, pay bills, and manage to show up to work once in a while. That was me. To the casual observer, I looked like the poster child for a working mother and devoted daughter. I was frequently asked that annoying question, "How do you do it all?" "One day at a time," I would answer with an offhand chuckle. But despite the upbeat façade, I was burned out. I was angry at my husband, who traveled for business, because he wasn't around to help more. I tried to hide my stress at work because the concept of "work-life balance" had not been discovered yet. But most of all, I was frustrated with myself for trying to be all things to too many people. Somehow, I was going to have to lower the bar and let things go. There just wasn't enough of me to go around.

Risks of Not Refueling

If you look up the term *burnout* in the Merriam-Webster dictionary, you will find the following definition: "the time when a jet or rocket engine stops working because there is not more fuel available." Applied to the human condition, burnout refers to "exhaustion of physical or emotional strength or motivation usually as a result of prolonged stress or frustration."[2] If we were all jet planes, we would simply put more fuel in our tanks and carry on, no worse for the wear. But we're not. We are complicated creatures who need more than just food and water to thrive in this world. As caregivers, our tanks may be depleted, but we keep going anyway. And eventually, we simply wear out our parts.

Dr. Barry J. Jacobs, author of *The Emotional Survival Guide for Caregivers: Looking After Yourself and Your Family While Helping an Aging Parent,* describes the typical signs of burnout as fatigue, irritability, sleeplessness, feelings of helplessness, and withdrawal from activities and social contacts.[3] Jacobs warns that isolated caregivers are particularly vulnerable to burnout and more at risk for depression. They cut themselves off from friends, family, and other supports because they don't have time for that stuff. They keep going until they can't anymore. And then what? They land in the emergency room with a herniated disc—or worse. Healthcare professionals try their best to intervene, but that may be after the damage is done.

Social Worker to the Rescue

As a social worker at a home health care agency, the referrals I received from the nurses had a similar theme. The family caregivers were barely holding on. Resources such as money, supportive siblings, and paid help always seemed to be in scarce supply. There was the adult daughter who had left her job to move in with her frail and chronically ill mother. Both women were lonely and depressed. There was the fifty-year-old man caring for his wife with metastatic cancer, overwhelmed with fear and grief, struggling to hold on to his job and raise his three kids. And I will never forget the daughter of a woman with chronic obstructive pulmonary disease who continued to sneak cigarettes, even though she needed oxygen therapy to breathe. One day, when the daughter left the house for an errand, her mother uncovered a hidden stash of cigarettes, lit one up, and set the house on fire.

One after the other, I heard their stories and did what I could to offer guidance and support. These caregivers felt frustrated and alone. I sympathized, humbled by their fortitude, courage, and vulnerability. But at the same time, I had no idea what it was like to be in their shoes. I was barely thirty years old. I had one child, a new home, and had not yet been tested by life's fragility. My world had just begun to expand. Yet, through the souls of these tired caregivers, I could see what happens when your world unexpectedly grows smaller. These people had relinquished a part of their being in order to care for someone else. They could barely carve out time to go the dentist, get a haircut, hang out with a friend—let alone care for themselves.

How could I, in my role as social worker, help them retrieve what had been lost? I wanted to throw out a lifeline and make meaningful recommendations within the two or three home visits most insurance plans allotted. I needed to offer tangible assistance without ignoring the emotional issues that impacted their well-being. Yes, there were concrete things I could offer from my grab bag of supports. I arranged for home health aides to pro-vide respite care, connected caregivers to local support groups, and found case management programs through the state home care agencies (now called Area Agencies on Aging). I helped one woman get a ramp installed so she did not have to literally lift her mother in a wheelchair to reach the car. Through the American Cancer Society, I found a volunteer to transport the woman with cancer to medical appointments, which provided some relief to her husband.

Although I was not able to wave my magic social worker wand and make it all better, I was able to make a modest difference. When people open themselves up to support and connection, change can occur and burdens can be lessened. I learned as much from these caregivers as they learned from me—important lessons that were helpful when I assumed a caregiving role within my own family. If you tip the scales toward too much self-sacrifice, you unknowingly put yourself and the person you care for at risk. You need to recognize that feeling overwhelmed and exhausted may be important signals that your system is on overload.

Somewhere between Selfless and Selfish

There's no way around it: caregiving is hard work and requires sacrifice. You signed on to a job without pay, promotions, a retirement plan, or long-term career growth. You may not even get paid the most important currency of caregiving—appreciation. Despite all your efforts, you may be denied the thanks you so richly deserve. You feel old. The halcyon days of your youth are behind you and you wistfully remember a time when you could do things on the spur of the moment without a care in the world. Now it seems like you have to plan every minute of every day. No wonder you feel a little sorry for yourself. Let's face it: caregiving can be fertile ground for self-pity. If you suffer from woe-is-me-itis, don't despair. There is help. Being selfless is all well and good—to a point. But sometimes being a little selfish allows you to care for yourself too.

As caregivers, we have the opportunity to connect to the better angels of our nature. When we are kind and compassionate, we feel good. When we are angry and guilt-ridden, we don't. To get through the murky emotional landscape of caregiving, we need to get real and embrace our inner Darth Vader. Yes, there will be days you feel grateful, but also times when you want to bop your loved one upside the head. Hugh Marriott's book *The*

Selfish Pig's Guide to Caring: How to Cope with the Emotional and Practical Aspects of Caring for Someone is a heartfelt and poignantly dark memoir of one man's long odyssey caring for his wife with Huntington's disease. Although the book focuses on the experience of being a "carer" in the United Kingdom, there are many universal themes that will resonate with caregivers elsewhere. Marriott talks bluntly about his isolation, guilt, and occasional murderous rage toward his chronically ill wife. He is an ordinary person who finds himself in a not-so-ordinary situation. He reacts as most people would and doesn't downplay the bad stuff. He gives voice to the unspeakable when he says, "It wasn't only me who came close to murder. Perhaps all carers did."[4]

Marriott, who cared for his wife for nine long years until her death, had some tools at his disposal to get through the arduous journey. His irreverent humor and gritty realism helped him cope with the range of emotions, both good and bad, that most caregivers experience along the way. Most people don't feel comfortable acknowledging the emotional underbelly of caregiving as bluntly at Marriott does. These darker emotions aren't a sign you're a bad person; they just mean you're human. But feelings of intense anger or frustration can be a warning sign too. If you feel like a powder keg, you may need a supportive person to confide in and a safe place to let off steam. If you're at the end of your rope, it may be time to step away from your caregiving duties, at least for a while, because you could be putting yourself and your loved one in harm's way.

Elder Abuse and Neglect

The vast majority of people, whether they are family members or professionals, take on caregiving for all the right reasons. They feel compassion, devotion, or a sense of gratification in helping others. But there are risks. Caregivers who run themselves into the ground may be more inclined to take it out on everyone around them, including their loved ones. When does this cross the line into harmful behavior? Can being stressed actually make you more prone to neglecting or abusing your loved one? How can you protect your elder and yourself from falling into this trap?

Each year, millions of older adults are abused or neglected. They suffer physical injury, emotional torment, and sexual assault at the hands of their caretakers. They are manipulated, deceived, and financially exploited. They are forgotten, ignored, and abandoned. *They* could be anyone—the next-door neighbor who keeps to himself or the popular celebrity adored by millions. At the age of ninety, Mickey Rooney, the vaudevillian actor and movie star, accused his stepchildren of emotional and financial abuse and denying him such basic necessities as food and medicine. His story shed light on the threat of elder abuse and neglect. How could adult children, whose role should be to care for and protect their parent, act with such greed and malice?

First, it's important to note that impatience, unkindness, and carelessness—all things that can result from frustration and stress—are not the same as thievery and assault. The notion that elder abuse is primarily caused by caregiver burnout and stress has generally been debunked.[5] Still, it happens. Some studies suggest that caregivers, especially those caring for a spouse with significant cognitive impairment and physical needs, are more likely to engage in harmful behavior.[6] In the case of financial exploitation, greed seems to be a big motivator. Many perpetrators of abuse strive to assert power and control over their victim, using tactics such as threats, intimidation, and manipulation. People with dementia are particularly vulnerable because they are less able to speak out against their abusers. As caregivers, we should pay attention to signs of abuse or neglect such as unexplained injuries, sudden fear of being bathed or changed, withdrawal, agitation, malnutrition, or unsanitary living conditions. If something doesn't feel right, trust your gut. Perhaps you have concerns about the home health aide, your parent's new "friend," or the long-lost relative who suddenly dotes on your mother. You may be the only person who will raise a red flag and take action. If you suspect someone you know or love is a victim of abuse or neglect, you should contact Adult Protective Services through your local Area Agencies on Aging or the National Adult Protective Services Association (www.napsa-now.org). You can confidentially report suspected elder abuse or neglect, which will trigger an investigation. What happens next? That depends on the circumstances and whether the alleged victim is willing to accept help. If not, there's not much that can be done. If the victim is willing to accept help, there is support available: housing resources, legal assistance, in-home care and, in more severe cases, court action to protect a victim from his or her abuser.

Although stress and anger may coexist with abusive behavior, they are not the cause. Most caregivers experience frustration, but very few intentionally abuse or neglect their loved ones. We love imperfectly. Some of us may even lose our cool and yell once in a while. As a harried mother, I often raised my voice a decibel or two when my kids were driving me crazy. I even got a T-shirt that said, "I yell because I care." When I found myself yelling more frequently over little things, it was a sign to stop and take care of myself. I called it my "Calgon, take me away" moment. Caregivers need those "take me away" moments and should not feel guilty about it. But those who most require a break often don't get one. These are typically caregivers providing over forty hours of care a week. They are less likely to seek help, at greater risk for burnout, and more likely to be a spouse. Sound familiar? Maybe you are worried about your dad, who is caring for your mom but not doing a very good job caring for himself. Or perhaps you are worried about yourself, caring for your life partner while trying to manage everything else. In my case it was my mom, caring for my dad. But she did figure out how to care for herself too. And that made all the difference.

Caring for Your Life Partner

Spousal caregivers, like my mother, are at particularly high risk. They often shoulder the physical burdens of caregiving and are more likely to experience financial strain.[7] Without proper support, spousal caregivers can face grave danger. They may be injured, fall, or get sick themselves. Those over the age of sixty-five have higher mortality rates than noncaregivers of the same age.[8] One of the reasons we chose to put my father in a nursing

home was to protect my mother. She'd suffered from repeated fractures due to osteoporosis, and after my father
became incontinent, she could not manage the heavy lifting and hands-on care. My mother was initially overcome
with guilt and sadness when my father's doctor recommended a nursing home. But over time she felt relief. "I
knew I couldn't handle him anymore," my mother explained. "And I was always aware of the importance of
taking care of myself. If I was not strong, I could not take
care of him."

How did she stay strong? She got help. She hired a
home health aide to do the bathing and dressing, and
found a volunteer who played cards and Parcheesi with
my dad. My father loved the added attention, and my
mother got a much-needed break. She joined a caregiver
support group through Jewish Family Services where she
could share her challenges and help others with theirs.
There, my mother met several women who were not adequately taking care of themselves. One woman was caring for both her mother and mentally ill brother on her
own, essentially giving up her life and wearing herself out.
Group members encouraged the woman to consider alternative care arrangements so she could free up space in
her life for herself too. Somehow, my mother managed to
do just that. During the twelve years of my father's illness,

my mother continued her work as a psychotherapist, had a strong circle of friends, and made time for visits to her children and grandchildren. Instead of feeling depleted, she felt fulfilled. There were difficult days, of course, when she deeply missed the man my father once was, and when she felt pained by his absence. But the imperative to remain strong was her guiding light and allowed my mother to care for my father with love and devotion until the end of his days.

What You Can Do

Caring for yourself when you are a caregiver is easier said than done. We start out with lofty intentions and believe we can manage it all. As time passes and demands pile up, we find ourselves gasping for air and searching for that oxygen mask to deploy. If you build in time to breathe, you'll be better able to pace yourself and less likely to fall into a self-defeating rut. Giving yourself a break can help you rejuvenate and, upon returning to caregiving, be ready to engage and connect in more fulfilling ways. Finding a network of support is crucial. You will need tangible help for sure, like home care, transportation, and expert guidance on what type of care to choose, but you'll also need to set aside time to nurture your soul. Men can be at a disadvantage here. They are less likely to reach out for emotional support, yet suffer from the same guilt and grief that women do. As my mother learned, feeling connected to a community of caregivers can make all the difference. Caregiver support groups can be found in most local hospitals and social service agencies. The Alzheimer's Association (www.alz.org) offers peer- and professionally led caregiver support groups facilitated by trained individuals. If you prefer a virtual experience, there are online options as well. The Family Caregiver Alliance (www .caregiver.org) offers a range of online groups that focus on Alzheimer's and dementia care, brain injuries, and the LGBT community.

If we don't want to run ourselves ragged, we also need to take care of our bodies in mindful and compassionate ways. For me, working out at the gym, taking a yoga class, or just going for a nice long WOG (combination walk/jog) keeps my mood in check and my body from creaking. We also need to pay attention to what we put into our bodies: food can either fuel or deplete us. If we skip meals or eat junk food, we'll pay a price. When I do that, my body sounds the alarm and I end up with a whopping migraine. Yes, it takes more time to eat a balanced, healthy diet, but doing so needs to be a habit, like a muscle, that you exercise and strengthen. And don't even think about catching up on emails by cutting back on sleep. Sleep is chicken soup for the body and the soul. If we walk around like sleep-deprived zombies, we won't be much help to anyone, least of all ourselves.

Spirituality and Self-Compassion

Many people find solace through some form of spiritual practice. Through ritual and a shared belief system, religious worship can provide a framework for caregivers to find comfort and compassion within a broader community. But there are other ways to nurture spirituality too. Taking a walk in the woods, listening to music, or writing in a journal may help you feel grounded in the present, rather than worrying about what's next. Meditation can give you a calmer and more positive connection with yourself and a practiced way to let your mind and body rest.

One of the most fundamental aspects of being an effective caregiver is to practice self-compassion. I spoke to Lisa Berzins, PhD, a clinical psychologist with thirty years of experience treating addictions and eating disorders. Berzins also teaches self-compassion as a form of healing. What is self-compassion? It's showing yourself the same kindness and care you would to a good friend. It's accepting your feelings without guilt or judgment and acknowledging your own pain. It's finding space within the broader human context of your experience for connection and compassion. In her clinical practice, Berzins uses the framework of self-compassion as a powerful tool to help people struggling with addiction and depression. It was also personally meaningful for Berzins, who describes herself as highly self-critical. "Self-compassion taught me to stop beating myself up and forgive my own mistakes," she acknowledged.

When caring for her father with dementia, Berzins found great relevance through the model of self-compassion. It helped her accept the bad and savor the good. That is our challenge as caregivers. If we ignore ourselves, we may not see what bounty this life has to offer. Berzins and I shared the experience of caring for a parent at times better than we cared for ourselves. We share something else too. Dr. Berzins is my sister. Together, we mourned the loss of my father and hold on dearly to his essence. When times are tough, my sister's words have been my guide: "May I be kind to myself and accept myself as I am. May I safely endure and make room for this pain. Only then can I truly experience life's joys."

ELEVEN

Letting Go

No one you love is ever truly lost.
—ERNEST HEMINGWAY

In one of my earliest memories of my father, I am three years old, during a vacation at Montauk Point on Long Island. We are walking along the beach when suddenly a foghorn makes a loud booming sound and I am terrified. Then my father holds me close, comforts me, and I feel protected and safe again. Three years later I am riding my bike home from Sunday school. I lose control over a patch of sand and go flying over the handlebars onto the pavement. I knock my tooth out, break my wrist, and have multiple cuts and bruises on my head and arms. I am just out of sight of my house—too dazed and injured to get up. Moments later, I see my father running toward me. He couldn't have seen my accident, yet somehow he knew something was wrong. Dad scoops me up and gets me to the hospital—my tooth is saved. To this day, I have no logical explanation for why my father dashed across the street when he did. I believe it was his innate intuition and deep empathic connection that enabled him to sense—in that moment, and many times throughout my life—that I needed him.

That intuition may have gone both ways. My very last visit with my father had not been planned. I remember having a sense that something was wrong, so I rearranged my weekend plans and drove to western Massachusetts to visit my dad. There was reason to be worried. After more than a decade with dementia, my father had weathered a particularly rough couple of months—bouncing in and out of the hospital with urinary tract infections. On more than one occasion, we thought the end was near. Somehow my father managed to pull through, always a bit worse for the wear. With each bout of illness he grew weaker and his tenacious hold on life seemed to be slipping away.

As soon as I entered his room at the nursing home I knew something was off. "Are you okay, Dad?" I asked. He shook his head no. "Are you in pain?" He nodded yes. I spoke to the nurse on duty, who said my father had seemed fine earlier in the day and had eaten a hearty lunch. That was typical. Even in the intensive care unit, my dad ate everything on his plate. But his appetite was not necessarily a barometer of his well-being. That would be the last thing to go. The nurse said she'd keep an eye on him and call if there was a problem. When I said good-bye, I gently kissed my father on the forehead. He tried his best to smile, but I could see the pain in his eyes.

At 2 a.m. the phone rang at my mother's house, where I was staying. My father had been in significant distress and was being transferred from the nursing home to the local hospital. We drove to the emergency room, somber, groggy, and frightened. There, my father rested on a hospital bed beneath the harsh lights. He had been sedated and looked at peace. The doctor explained that my father had a perforated bowel and it would not be long. We stayed for a while, then decided to return to my mother's house for a few hours of rest before returning to the hospital. As we pulled into the hospital parking lot several hours later, my mother's cell phone rang. It was the attending physician delivering the grim news. Minutes earlier, my father had died. My mother let out a gut-wrenching wail and I began to sob. Mixed in with our grief was a sense of guilt, because we hadn't been there to say good-bye.

Grief and Guilt

Anyone who has cared for a loved one with dementia knows that the grieving process begins long before the person actually dies. We witness the disease slowly robbing its victims of their capacities. It's called the "long good-bye." We anticipate the loss and steel ourselves for the emotional sucker punch we know is coming. But are we ever really ready to let go? Given his long, slow decline, the news of my father's death did not come as a shock. Still—it brought a wave of grief that I had not fully anticipated, followed by an overwhelming sense of guilt. Why hadn't we stayed in the hospital so we could have been there when he died? Did we do enough to alleviate my father's suffering in the end? Guilt, our constant companion as caregivers, emerges with renewed force upon a loved one's death. No matter how much we do, there's the nagging feeling that we could have done more. Accepting our limitations as caregivers and acknowledging that we are not saviors is part of the process of letting go.

In his final days, it was my father who was finally ready to let go. The week before he died, he let us know that he was ready to give up the fight. "This is too much," he said to my mother, as the smile that had so often graced his face was replaced by a dull resignation. Those somber words heralded the end was near and the grief we had anticipated for so long would soon enshroud us.

When I learned about the stages of grief at Simmons School of Social Work, from denial to acceptance, I imagined a linear process in which people completed one emotional task, then moved on to the next. The reality of grieving is far more complex. Mourning comes in waves, retreats gradually, and then resurfaces with unannounced intensity. During a trip to the bank months after my father died, I observed a woman take a lollipop for her daughter. I remembered how I would bring my father lollipops as a forbidden treat that he would relish with childlike glee during my many visits to the nursing home. As I imagined him enjoying the candy, I began to cry. The memory triggered the pain of my father's loss, but despite the sadness, it also brought a smile to my face.

As we move through the grieving process, we may be helped along, as my family was, by rituals and religious practices that bind us together and bring us comfort within the broader context of a community. After my father's funeral, we observed Shiva—the seven days of mourning practiced in the Jewish faith. I was deeply moved by the embrace of friends, who stocked my freezer with chicken, bagels, casseroles, and cakes. I regaled them with anecdotes about my father that revealed his unusual ability to use humor and imagination to cope with years of dementia and decline. I laughed as I retold my father's corny jokes—even his remark, each time we drove past a cemetery, "People are dying to get in there." And I remember something else too. As I spoke about my father, my friends who had lost parents, even decades earlier, began to tear up. Their sense of loss, though diminished by time, was still palpable. The grieving process, with its messy jumble of emotions, continues long after our loved ones are gone.

Earned Relief

There may be a hole in your heart after the death of a parent, but don't be shocked if you feel some relief too. Caregivers are often hesitant to acknowledge this relief for fear of being seen as selfish or uncaring. But according to Barry Jacobs, a clinical psychologist and family therapist, relief is normal—and often earned.[1] The weary work of caregiving requires a great deal of sacrifice and takes a toll, especially on spousal caregivers who are always on call. There's a reason for the notion of the merry widow. The end of caregiving may lead to new beginnings and an opportunity to explore other life pursuits. That is how my mother felt. She was deeply saddened by my father's death, but relieved his suffering was finally over. Knowing she had done her best helped to assuage those pangs of guilt caregivers so often experience. By the time my father died, my mother had been a caregiver for over twelve years. She had had the opportunity to prepare for the end, and anticipating the loss made it easier to accept when the time came.

A Rapid Decline

For others, the end is more abrupt and the grieving process feels like it's on fast-forward. That was the case with Reena, who was very close to her mother Esther, whom she described as the "Energizer bunny." In July, Esther, hale and hearty, was zip-lining in Costa Rica. By September, she was emaciated, unable to walk, and rapidly wasting away from multiple myeloma. Just sixty-five, Esther had survived breast cancer and reached the five-year mark—hoping to finally breathe a sigh of relief. But that was not to be. "I did everything right," Esther said. She was a yoga enthusiast, ate a healthy diet, and maintained an optimistic attitude despite all she'd endured. Why was this happening again? Reena, the oldest of three children and the only daughter, was the point person for her mother's care. She meticulously kept track of everything: expenses, medication, doctor's appointments, and volunteer drivers from the Cancer Society. This hyper-organization helped Reena manage her anxiety and gave her some sense of control over a difficult and disruptive situation.

For Reena, being communicator-in-chief felt like a burden too. Esther frequently directed medical questions at Reena, even though one of her sons was an oncologist. "Why not ask Stew?" Reena suggested to her mother one day. "I don't want to bother him. He's busy," Esther replied. "And I'm not?" Reena, a mother of two and a full-time human resource manager, did not have a lot of free time, so she had to be resourceful. There were tools that could help Reena and her family get through this ordeal, such as CaringBridge (www.caringbridge.org), a free and secure website that provides an online community of care. CaringBridge allowed Reena to post updates about Esther's condition and to receive ongoing support from family and friends. "Not only was it a huge time-saver," said Reena, "but those words of encouragement and love kept me going."

To Tell the Truth

In the hospital, Esther repeatedly answered questions from doctors and medical residents who paraded in and out of her room on a daily basis. Yet with all this information, no one seemed to be telling Esther the truth—that no amount of chemo would save her from a disease that was rapidly taking her life. Then one day, a second-year oncology fellow came by to check on Esther. Unlike some of the other doctors, he did not seem to be in a rush. He had a soft-spoken, gentle manner and a direct way of talking, without spouting euphemisms or averting his gaze. He did not suggest new drug trials or experimental treatments. He knew they had passed that point. Instead, the doctor asked Esther what she wanted, what mattered to her, and how she wanted to spend her remaining time.

In his book *Being Mortal: Medicine and What Matters in the End*, Dr. Atul Gawande, a physician and best-selling author, talks about the healthcare system's primary focus on ensuring survival for as long as possible.[2] Yet when our mortal bodies break down from debility and disease, can prolonging life lead to more harm than good? Gawande argues that it can. He believes that physicians, not wanting to dispel a patient's desperate hope for a cure, may offer treatments that are not likely to work and may even increase suffering. Gawande claims that the job of caring institutions is not to prolong life at all costs but to enable well-being. That means physicians need to have conversations about end of life care to give people like Esther the right information to decide how best to spend their final days.

If you talk to doctors nowadays, you'll find many of them are not all that happy. Data entry demands from electronic medical records can encroach on precious time to actually talk to patients. And discussing death and dying? Not only has that been a topic to avoid, it's been a much-maligned one too. Remember "death panels"? But there is some good news out there, not just for the beleaguered docs, but also for the patients and families who need straight and compassionate talk about end of life. And it's coming from an unlikely source: Medicare. In 2016, Medicare began covering advance care planning—discussions that physicians and healthcare professionals can have with their patients about end of life care—as a separate billable service.[3] These are purely voluntary conversations that may open the door for options to increase quality of life in the end.

Hospice and Palliative Care

Over the years that I've worked in senior care, not once have I heard anyone wish they'd waited a little longer before they chose hospice. In fact, the opposite is more often true. Why do people typically avoid this type of care? For many, it feels like they are giving up the fight. And while choosing hospice is an acknowledgment that your days are numbered (and that number is usually six months or less), those days may be better spent at home with hospice, surrounded by family, rather than languishing away in a hospital bed.

Hospice care offers a holistic model in which physicians, nurses, social workers, home health aides, spiritual counselors, and volunteers work together to provide compassionate care and support to terminally ill patients and their families. Like Esther, people often put off the decision to seek hospice care. Many people receive hospice for a much shorter time than the six months typically allowed under their insurance benefit. In fact, half of terminally ill patients in the United States receive hospice care for less than three weeks, and one-third die within seven days.[4] No wonder: we live in a death-denying culture where even the word *hospice* conjures up the grim reaper. People of color are particularly reticent to seek out hospice care.[5] Cultural taboos, mistrust of the health-care system, and the pressure on families to assume the lion's share of caregiving may be factors. Yet, as terminally ill people better understand their options, hospice may become more compelling. In most cases hospice is provided in the home, but it can also be offered in institutional settings such as hospice centers, nursing homes, hospitals, and long-term care facilities. Hospice is one of the most comprehensive benefits covered by Medicare, with a focus on caring rather than curing. That may be a hard pill to swallow at first, but it's a beneficial option for many people struggling with a terminal disease. Hospice's model of pain and symptom management is designed to help people choose how they want to live, no matter how short their time may be.

People are often confused about the difference between hospice and palliative care. Like hospice, palliative care offers an interdisciplinary approach of symptom management administered through a single program. Unlike hospice, however, palliative care is available to anyone who has a serious illness, not just the terminally ill.[6] It is the bridge between acute medical treatment and end of life hospice care. Hospice relies heavily on family caregivers in the home, like Reena, whereas palliative care is typically delivered by doctors, nurses, and other medical professionals in hospitals and healthcare institutions. Opting for hospice care means foregoing aggressive curative treatment, a decision Esther eventually made. She wanted to spend her remaining time enjoying what mattered most: her children and grandchildren. Reena decided it was best to take her mother home, to her house, surrounded by the chaos of children, a ten-year-old Rottweiler, a pet hamster named Skippy, and a whole lot of love.

A Good Death

Karen Mannal, a nurse practitioner, knows firsthand the value of hospice. "Patients and families are profoundly grateful for the care and support," Mannal explains. "We would ask our patients: what would make each day as good as it could be? If the patient loved music, we'll play them music. If they like to laugh, we're going to tell jokes. One woman said her favorite food was pizza. So we got her a pepperoni pizza smothered in cheese. She took one bite, which was all she could manage, and smiled."

Enabling people to die as peacefully as possible, relatively free from pain, in a supported and dignified manner is one of the primary goals of hospice. When Esther passed away, she did not appear to be suffering, and seemed comforted by the presence of her children as she took her last breath. But, according to Mannal, the actual process of dying does not always resemble the bedside death depicted in many Hollywood movies. In her documentary film *This American Death*, Susan Austin, filmmaker and family caregiver, tells the story of her experience caring for her mother, who died of lung cancer.[7] Austin became preoccupied with the notion of "a good death"—the image of your loved one painlessly drifting out of this life surrounded by family and friends. After bearing witness to her mother's agonizing illness, Austin concludes that the process of dying can be unpredictable and frightening for caregivers. Having support is crucial, both during and after a loved one's death.

Mannal agrees. "Some people lash out as they are dying, get extremely anxious, and become unrecognizable to their family members." This can be tough for caregivers and may exacerbate simmering disagreements about what's best for a loved one. Family members may take opposing sides and engage in intractable conflicts that may last years after the death of a parent—even generations if not resolved. All the forces that pull us apart and hold us together come roaring to the surface as we face difficult decisions regarding death and dying. Hospice strives to get family members on the same page as much as possible: to support the dying person and each other. But what steps can you take ahead of time to pave the way for the inevitable and do what's best for your loved ones—and yourself?

Discussing Death with a Cup of Joe

Does the idea of hanging out with a group of strangers sipping decaf latte and schmoozing about death sound appealing? Apparently it does to some. Death cafés are not a new Starbucks spin-off designed to capture the aging demographic market share. No, this is a grassroots movement started by a web designer in London who had a crazy notion. He thought bringing people together to dish about death while drinking hot potables might be a good idea. Death is one of those subjects people assiduously avoid. But there seems to be some collective benefit from sharing profound questions and universal fears about this taboo topic in a casual and open forum. Apparently the idea has taken hold and there are over forty countries that now host death cafés. Who knows? You may find one in your neck of the woods (www.deathcafe .com).

Talking about death can be a good starting point for planning ahead. There are some practical steps to take that can make decisions about end of life care less agonizing for everyone. The first is to explore and understand your loved one's wishes. Imagine—you're waiting in the emergency room with your father, who is mentally incapacitated, and the physician asks, "Is there a DNR (do not resuscitate) order?" When faced with the urgency of a life-or-death decision, your heart and your head may be out of sync. I should know, because the man in the emergency room was my dad. In that moment, my heart won out and I said no to the DNR. But upon reflection, after the crisis, my family and I determined that a DNR was the right choice and putting my father through an agonizing ordeal to extend his life would not be what he wanted. No one wants to think about this stuff. But engaging in meaningful conversations about what to do if . . . may give you a much-needed compass when the time comes. Fortunately, a website exists that guides us through this process: The Conversation Project (www.theconversationproject.org). The website even provides a starter kit that outlines how to kick-start the conversation, what to ask, and how to keep it straightforward and simple.

Tough Topics

These sensitive and highly personal conversations should be taking place initially in kitchens and living rooms rather than in hospitals. But bringing up death and dying with your parents or elders may be something we avoid precisely because it is fraught with emotional land mines. Roz Chast, in her hilarious and heart-wrenching graphic memoir, *Can't We Talk about Something More Pleasant?*, illustrates the frustration of trying to confront an issue that her parents are determined to avoid.[8] Chast, an only child, assumes the punishing task of caring for her parents, who both lived into their nineties and refused to acknowledge or discuss their own decline. In the end, Chast's mother languished near death far longer than expected, defying the predictions of her hospice caregivers. What Chast's mother did express, which wasn't much to go on, was that she did not want her life prolonged, only to become a lump of "pulsating protoplasm."

My own mother made it much easier on my siblings and me. Following the guidelines of The Conversation Project, we had an honest discussion about what she might want. It's a hard topic to think about, though my mother's just shy of ninety and has endured a number of serious illnesses and injuries. Despite all that, she is a bundle of energy and, at the age of eighty-seven, reluctantly retired from her long-standing psychotherapy practice. When it came to discussing what she would want, my mother made it pretty clear. She did not want artificial or heroic measures to keep her alive, assuming there was no hope for recovery. "Let nature take its course," she said. To understand more, we discussed how much she'd like to be told about her health condition (everything) and with whom she would want this information shared (close friends and family). We explored what type of setting she'd prefer to receive care in if she was terminally ill (home, if possible). And most important, my mother didn't want us to fight about anything. "If anybody really wants a piece of furniture, artwork, or jewelry, let me know now because I don't want you arguing about it when I'm dead," she said matter-of-factly.

Put It in Writing

Even with proactive conversations, end of life wishes can be misunderstood and subject to interpretation. That's why it's important to capture this information in writing and have an advanced directive such as a healthcare proxy. Also referred to as a durable power of attorney for healthcare, a healthcare proxy is a simple document that can be obtained from your doctor's office or even downloaded off the Internet. When you draft a healthcare proxy, you name a trusted person, usually a family member, as your designated agent, responsible for carrying out your wishes and making medical decisions if you can't make them yourself. My mother appointed my older sister Lisa as her healthcare proxy. Lisa will have the tough task of making medical decisions (with help from me and my brother) based, of course, on what my mother wants. What about finances? Tag, I'm it. As the designated durable power of attorney (POA) for financial matters, I will need to figure out how to pay bills and manage the money. This is all part of my mother's will, which thankfully she did on her own, without prompting or nagging from her children. That is not always the case. Roz Chast's parents did not have a will until they were in their nineties, and by then, they were not in such great shape. Yes, death and dying are not pleasant subjects to discuss, but planning ahead can eliminate the guesswork and lay the groundwork for what's most important in the end.

Holding on While Letting Go

After we received the news that my father had died, we grimly proceeded to his hospital room, where my dad lay motionless, his body still warm. It was a gruesome sight and we cried out from horror and grief. The hospital staff did not rush us and instead let me and my family take the time we needed to say our good-byes. That turned out to be a gift. We stayed for hours and found comfort in talking to my father, knowing he could not hear us, but realizing he was still very present in our lives.

After losing a parent, we build a nest within our heart—and find a place to hold their memory. That is how we hold on, while still letting go. We strive to honor their legacy and we may do this in a number of different ways. My brother made a film about my father, telling the story of his life, before and after dementia. My sister gave a presentation to mental health providers on dementia and self-compassion. My mother is currently writing her memoir, a legacy she will pass on to her grandchildren so they will know their history. I encourage family members to take the time, before it is too late, to capture the intricate stories and life lessons we've learned and witnessed, so our parents will live on in our memories long after they are gone. The death of a parent is a stark reminder that our time will come. Yet it is precisely this knowledge that helps us savor what we have, the people in our lives who are still with us, and the ones, like my father, who live on in our souls.

TWELVE

Moving Forward, Looking Back

I want to turn the clock back to when people lived in
small villages and took care of each other.
—PETE SEEGER

Benjamin Franklin once said that the only things certain
in life are death and taxes. But if you ask some visionary
entrepreneurs, death might possibly be "cured" one day.
Even if Silicon Valley can figure out how to hack the code
of life, would cheating death rob us of what really matters
in life? I'll leave that to the philosophy majors to debate.
Despite unprecedented increases in the human life span,
eventually we'll all make our final exit from this world. As
explained by Rafiki, the baboon narrator of *The Lion King*,
it's the circle of life. And as we grow old and our bodies

start to wear down, a good number of us are going to need help along the way. Looking ahead—who is going to provide that care? What will it look like? Will we rely on technology to fill the gaps? And what are the uniquely human lessons we learn as caregivers that, despite new trends on the horizon, are timeless?

The Looming Caregiver Shortage

When it comes to the growing demand for caregiving, the numbers just don't add up. The United States, like many industrialized countries, is looking down the barrel of a looming care gap. As my fellow baby boomers move headlong into old age, there may not be enough caregivers to go around. The potential pool of family caregivers, those devoted daughters and sons whose stories I have told throughout this book, is rapidly dwindling. An estimated 117 million Americans will need assistance of some kind by 2020, yet the number of unpaid caregivers is expected to reach only 45 million.[1] The caregiver support ratio, the number of potential family caregivers relative to the number of older Americans, is projected to decline sharply by midcentury.[2] Where have all the caregivers gone? Declining birth rates, far-flung families, a rising number of women in the workforce, and the projected increase in Alzheimer's disease and dementia are contributing to this supply/demand conundrum. The responsibility of caring for a growing population of seniors will be borne by fewer family members. Now more than ever, this diminishing but not diminished army of caregivers needs to prepare for what lies ahead.

Many will seek to hire paid caregivers, who will be increasingly in demand as the population ages. Only about three in ten older adults who require daily assistance hire paid caregivers now. But that percentage may increase, since there won't be enough family members to go around.[3] The U.S. Bureau of Labor Statistics estimates that nursing assistants and home health aides are among the top ten occupations with the greatest projected job growth in the United States. These unsung heroes, who are disproportionately women of color, work for low wages and are often economically powerless.[4] They are people like Roseline, a home health aide who tenderly cared for my father during the last years of his life and always greeted him with a hug and a smile. She bathed and dressed him and tended to my father's needs with skill and compassion. She performed a job that our society does not sufficiently reward.

How can we help people like Roseline, part of a vital care workforce, who often live below the poverty line, dependent upon public assistance to support their families? Fortunately, there are industry leaders and innovators who are taking a stand and pushing for change. In 2010, Ai Jen Poo, the executive director of the NDWA (National Domestic Workers Alliance), helped lead the passage of the Domestic Workers Bill of Rights, the first in the United States to guarantee domestic workers basic labor protections, signed into law in a growing number of states. And entrepreneurs like Sheila Lirio Marcelo, founder, chairwoman, and CEO of Care.com, the world's largest online marketplace for finding and managing care, are committed to addressing the complex care challenges that impact families. "There needs to be a culture change in how we perceive care workers, who are essential to our ability to work and manage our lives," Marcelo says. In 2015, Care.com and NDWA helped launch the "Fair Care Pledge," a national effort advocating for fair pay, paid time off, and clear job responsibilities for professional caregivers, so they can continue to provide the help families so desperately need.

But if wages for paid caregivers do increase, as they should, how will the average family afford care? Most families are digging deep into their pockets already. Will public policy offer some type of relief? Maybe, but don't hold your breath. The national uncertainty over healthcare policy is only making matters worse. Legislative gridlock may be one of the things we can count on in life, up there with death and taxes.

There are, however, a number of worthy public policy initiatives trying to make their way through Congress. Take the Social Security Caregiver Credit Act, for instance, which would provide Social Security credit for caregivers of dependent elders and children who have to leave the workforce. Or the FAMILY Act, which would offer up to twelve weeks of partial income to those eligible for FMLA (Family Medical Leave Act), already provided in some states. How about a little tax relief? The Credit for Caring Act would provide a tax credit of up to $3,000 for qualified families to help defray the cost of caring for a loved one. It may be a drop in the bucket, but every little bit helps.

While the growing financial burden of long-term care looms large, attempts to create a safety net to cover the cost of that care have not always made it to the finish line. The failure of the CLASS Act (Community Living Assistance Services and Support) is one example. The brainchild of the late Senator Ted Kennedy, the CLASS Act would have provided a voluntary and public long-term insurance care option for people anticipating the cost of their own care one day. Unfortunately, it met its demise in 2011, when it was repealed before it even got off the ground. Perhaps family caregivers need to band together and launch a social movement. It may be time to stage a million caregivers march so our voices are heard and action finally taken.

There is plenty of uncertainty on the horizon. Will Medicare, which faces an ominous threat of insolvency, take on the burgeoning costs of long-term care? Will Medicare even be around when all those millennials start turning sixty-five? What about Medicaid? How about expanding programs that cover home- and community-based services to keep more frail elders out of costly nursing homes? And the caregiving workforce? Will folks like Roseline leave their jobs altogether and find higher-paying work elsewhere? Perhaps wages for paid caregivers will naturally rise as demand outstrips supply. And that leaves us all with a challenge—how will we pay for long-term care when our time comes? You can't necessarily rely on the government for help, so it's best to plan ahead. As Theodore Roosevelt once said, "Aging is like anything else. To make a success of it, you've got to start young."

Home Sweet Home

Most people as they approach old age are going to want to live out their golden years as independently as possible —staying connected to the things they know and love.

According to Laurie Orlov, founder and principal analyst of Aging in Place Technology Watch, a consultancy on technology for seniors, most older adults will choose to live in their homes until they can't anymore. Orlov says that the current trend in eldercare is away from institutional care and more focused on aging in place. And technology is likely to play an increasingly important role in keeping people safe at home. Many technological solutions that ease the burden of caregiving are available now, but adoption has been slow. Why? Barriers include privacy concerns, cost (often not covered by insurance), and the fact that caregivers just don't have time to try new things. But younger generations, like the 75 million millennials heading en masse toward the ranks of caregivers, are particularly adept and comfortable with tech-based solutions for just about everything—from finding a date to caring for Mom.

Should my kids need to take care of me and my husband, they will have all sorts of technology options at their disposal—a caregiving version of *The Jetsons*. Even if they live halfway around the planet, remote activity monitoring through in-home sensors can alert them to worrisome changes in our daily routines. I'm not sure I want my son to know I spent an unusual amount of time in the bathroom one Tuesday, but it may be worth it if the technology allows me to stay put in my home. What if we don't remember to take our pills? There are plenty of options to help with that too. Dispensers with remote monitoring can notify family caregivers as to whether meds have been taken, and devices like Reminder Rosie can record customized prompts. Rather than listening to a generic beep, perhaps my musical daughter can remind me to take my weekly osteoporosis pill with a tune—a little ditty combining tones and bones.

In the future, technology is likely to help with many of the caregiving challenges we now face. Your father can't drive anymore? Why not order a self-driving car to take him to the senior center? Your mother's fallen and can't get up? Her wearable device can signal emergency responders (and you) that she needs help. That nifty wristband may also monitor vital signs, keep track of doctor visits, send alerts if she's inactive, and suggest a meditation exercise when she's stressed. But nothing seems more like a brave new world than robot caregivers. These mechanical creatures are rapidly becoming more sophisticated, although for now they are still too costly for the average person to consider. Don't have time to do Mom's laundry, mop the floor, or remind her to take Lyrica? Let R2-D2 do it. You don't have to worry that Robot will burn out or need time off for vacation, sick leave, or even sleep. And if your dad is feeling a bit lonely—maybe Robot can read him his favorite book or greet him when he wakes up in the morning. Some nursing homes are even turning to robotic therapy pets to calm the agitation and anxiety caused by dementia.[5] A robotic cat made by Hasbro, called Joy for All Companion Pets, requires no Fancy Feast or kitty litter. While research about the lasting benefits of animatronic pets is inconclusive, the proof may be in the petting.

So, with all this technology, will family caregivers still be needed in a highly connected, tech-enabled world? Despite mind-blowing advances in artificial intelligence, people will probably always need people. The vital importance of human connection, in my opinion, will never be replaced by a machine or an algorithm. After all, caring for another human being, with all its contradictions and complexities, is about love. So long as we are alive, the ability to give and receive love can persevere, and neither illness nor decline can extinguish it. As our once strong parents grow old, they suffer loss, yet they continue to love us as we continue to love them. These familial bonds are powerful and lasting and can pass from one generation of caregivers to the next.

Lasting Gifts

Back in the 1970s, when my parents insisted that my siblings and I visit my grandmother in the nursing home, I initially felt resentful about this onerous responsibility. At age fifteen, I had better things to do—or so I thought—than hang out with a bunch of scary-looking old people. But at some point something changed, and to my surprise, I started to look forward to those visits. My "senile" grandmother Bubbie, who by then spoke a mishmash of five languages, always lit up when I arrived. She would smile, tenderly caress my hand, and refer to me as Bubeleh ("dear one" in Yiddish). At the same time, I also got to know some of the other residents at the nursing home. Once I did, they became real people whose rich and interesting life stories could be uncovered if you only took the time to ask. I particularly remember Edna and Fred, a frail old couple who had been married for sixty years, which seemed like an eternity to my fifteen-year-old mind. They had two children (one who had died in childhood) and several grandchildren. But I rarely saw them with visitors, and they seemed happy to adopt me as their surrogate granddaughter. One day when I came to visit Bubbie, I saw Edna slumped in a chair by herself. Just two days earlier, Fred had suffered a stroke and died. I cried when I heard the news. I wasn't sure what to say or do to comfort someone in mourning, but I made it a point to include Edna during my many visits to Bubbie. While I didn't know it at the time, Bubbie and Edna had taught me an important lesson about the power of connection, which I would teach my own children one day, when I too would become a caregiver.

While there is tremendous focus on the burdens of caregiving, of which there are many, there is less attention paid to the numerous benefits. A study by the National Opinion Research Center revealed that 83 percent of family caregivers surveyed viewed it as a positive experience.[6] Over the many dozens of interviews I conducted for this book, I found this to be true, even among those whose experiences were the most burdensome. Many report feeling deeply gratified that they were able to give back and make a difference in their parents' lives. Others reflect upon the unexpected gifts of caregiving—the shift in perspective that often crystallizes what's important in life.

One woman, who described times when she cared for her mother as "hellish," recognized all that she had gained years later. "The best thing that ever happened to me was caring for my mother. It gave me humility and patience. It was a growth path for me and gave me character and fortitude. And it ultimately made me appreciate much more about life." Andy, who moved his 102-year-old grandmother to live with him, his wife, and four children, expressed a similar sentiment. "My grandmother had wisdom and a groundedness that was remarkable. She was kind, had a good sense of humor, and appreciated being part of the family." Caring for his grandmother often required a shift of attention away from his children. But Andy accepted the trade-off. "Overall, it was a net positive for sure, and my kids learned a valuable lesson about what it means to care for another person."

Some people feel that when they positively model caregiving, their children will grow up to be more compassionate human beings. I like to think that is true. My father's decline started while my children were still young, so they never really knew him in his prime. As a result of their visits, each one of my children made a special effort to engage with my dad during the many years of his dementia. My father loved seeing them and they saw and loved his warm, sweet personality. As my father's dementia deepened and his passivity grew, my children had the experience of working harder to reach him, and periodically drawing him out of his shell. When they successfully managed to reach through the fog, my father would show flashes of his brilliant, irreverent, mischievous personality —to their astonishment and delight.

It was my daughter Rebecca who forged the most pro-found bond with my father. Perhaps it was her beautiful singing that broke through the barrier to communication posed by dementia. Or perhaps she sensed my father's pain more acutely because she too felt wounded and di-minished during the tumultuous years of her adolescence. Reflecting back, Rebecca describes the lasting impact of her connection to my father: "When I visited my grand-father, my best self came forward. My efforts to find his light brightened my own. He taught me to look hard for the humanity in people, in all people, including those we might be inclined to dismiss. Someone who seemed like he was far gone actually had this vibrant self with an ac-tive imagination, swirling with pieces of lucidity and mys-tery. What a shame to miss out on that."

A dear friend, whose husband succumbed to an ago-nizing battle with cancer, said that from this heartrend-ing experience she learned what's most important. Before he died, my friend's husband told her the three things he needed most: to be seen, to be heard, and to be held. She took some comfort in knowing that she was able to give him those. While it sounds simple, a depth of emo-tional presence is required to make that happen. It is the fundamental essence of caregiving. It was what Rebecca provided my father and what he, in turn, gave back to her. It is what my mother modeled for my siblings and me during her twelve-year odyssey caring for my dad. There is so much that we as caregivers do to help our parents, hold them, and make them feel seen and understood. In return, caring for our parents teaches us to shoulder our sorrows and become intimate with our own inner strengths. The burdens and benefits of caregiving are what make up the richly woven fabric of this profound life experience. As we certainly encounter hurdles, may we also cherish the rewards: a sweet smile of appreciation, a warm embrace, and the unexpected gift that our efforts as caregivers will enrich the lives of those we love—and our own lives as well.

Tips and Checklists

Adapted from content courtesy of Care.com

A Proactive Approach to Caregiving

- **Have conversations early:** No one wants to talk about needing care one day, but it's better to understand your parents' preferences before a crisis occurs. Start by saying you want what's best for them and show concern for their safety and well-being, should they need help down the road.

- **Observe changes:** Have you or your siblings noticed changes in your parents' behavior, functioning, and mood? If so, discuss your observations and concerns together, then decide how best to approach your parents. Try to obtain a definitive medical diagnosis, from a geriatrician if possible, so you can explore appropriate options for care.

- **Read up:** Learn about different types of care, such as in-home care, adult day programs, nursing homes, and assisted living communities.

Attend a seminar or webinar about caregiving and aging offered by your employer or local senior care organization.

- **Explore finances:** Does your father have money stashed away to pay for long-term care? Does he have long-term care insurance, Medicaid, or veterans benefits? To avoid pitfalls, learn ahead of time about the cost of care and how it is paid for.

- **Get your documents in order:** Has a health-care proxy been appointed for someone to make health-related decisions should your father become incapacitated? Have consent forms been signed to allow family members to communicate with the medical team? Are legal documents in place, such as a power of attorney, to enable someone to manage financial matters if your parent is unable to do so?

- **Seek out expert advice:** The assistance of a social worker, care manager, elder law attorney, or financial advisor can go a long way in guiding you through the legal, financial, and emotional challenges of caregiving.

When Your Parent Refuses Help

- **Start early:** Bring up the topic of long-term care when your parent is still active and healthy. That way, you'll have a framework for putting a plan in place if and when the time comes.

- **Recruit an outsider:** It may take an outside voice (or two) to get your mother to agree to help. Recruit doctors, healthcare professionals, and family members to persuade Mom to accept the care she needs.

- **Take it slowly:** If possible, slowly integrate a paid caregiver into your father's routine. Have the caregiver come a couple times a week to help with laundry and food prep, then gradually increase the number of visits, if needed. Giving your dad time to develop a positive relationship with a care provider may enable him to accept help on his own terms.

- **Don't take away control:** Respecting a parent's autonomy and right to make decisions, even bad ones, may be a hard pill to swallow. But insisting parents accept help or else usually backfires. Avoid admonitions and use a calm, empathic approach as much as possible.

- **Accept your limits:** If, despite all your efforts, your mother still says no, there may be little else you can do. Your ability to take care of someone who doesn't accept help is limited, and you still need to find time to take care of yourself.

Home Dangers Every Caregiver Should Know

- **Poor lighting:** Many seniors have some degree of vision impairment. Make sure walkways, hallways, and stairs are well lit—inside and out.

- **Clutter:** Note if things are piled up on the stairs, by the door, or on the counters too near (or even on) the stove. Be aware of clutter on shelves and in upper cabinets that can fall and cause injury.

- **Fall risks:** Slippery throw rugs, loose carpet, and uneven floor surfaces can pose a tripping hazard. Extension cords, wires, and cables should be positioned out of the flow of foot traffic.

- **Bath and water hazards:** Adjust the water heater to a safe maximum of 120 degrees. Place nonskid mats in front of the sink and tub to absorb excess water and prevent falls. Consider a tub/shower combo that has a step and molded seat, or a sit-in

shower. Install grab bars next to the toilet and
around the tub.

- **Food and fire hazards:** Is food stored properly,
and has expired food been thrown out? Are burn-
ers or the oven ever left on? Are smoke detectors
and carbon monoxide detectors properly installed
and up to date? Consider getting rid of candles
and space heaters, which can be fire hazards.

- **Home temperature:** Is the house too cold or too
hot? Set the thermostat at a consistent, comfortable temperature. You can also install climate control technology so you can adjust the thermostat
remotely from your smart phone.

- **Car safety:** Are there unexplained dents on the
car? Are the auto insurance and registration up to
date? Can your mother open the garage door
manually if she needs to? Explore whether there
are alternative means of transportation available if
your parent can no longer drive.

- **Communication:** Are there various ways to
reach your mother, including a cell phone, land-
line, and Skype? Ask for names of neighbors or
friends whom you can contact in an emergency.
If your mom is at risk for falls, consider a medical
alert system so she can quickly access help in an
emergency.

Paying for Long-Term Care

Learn the basics about payer options such as Medicare, Medicaid, long-term care insurance, and veterans benefits.

Medicare is health insurance administered by the federal government for people sixty-five and over, younger adults with certain disabilities, and those with end-stage renal disease. Medicare covers a wide range of health-related expenses but typically does not cover long-term care.

Medicare has four parts:

- **Part A:** Covers most medically necessary hospital expenses, limited care in a skilled nursing facility, home health, and hospice.
- **Part B:** Covers doctors' visits, medical tests, outpatient hospital costs, physical therapy, rehabilitation, and some medical equipment.

- **Part C:** Offered through private health insurance plans, Medicare benefits called Medicare Advantage Plans include Parts A and B and sometimes prescription drug coverage.
- **Part D:** Provides prescription drug coverage. There can be a gap in coverage, referred to as the "donut hole," when Medicare recipients are responsible for the full cost of drugs up to a certain threshold.

Medicaid is a joint federal and state program that funds medical costs based on income eligibility. Medicaid benefits and eligibility vary by state, but most recipients cannot have more than $2,000 in assets or must "spend down" medical expenses to meet this threshold. Unlike Medicare, Medicaid will pay for long-term care such as a nursing home for those impaired enough to qualify.

Veterans Administration benefits, U.S. Department of Veterans Affairs: Offered to veterans and their spouses. Veterans eligible for a VA pension who are either housebound or require the care of another person may qualify for the aid and attendance benefit, which can pay for care at home or in a nursing home.

Long-term care insurance: A type of private insurance that provides limited coverage (often after an initial waiting period) for long-term care. Prices vary depending on the type of plan as well as the age and health status of the policyholder.

Seek Workplace Support

- **Flexible schedule:** Inquire about flexible hours or "flextime," which may help you better balance caregiving and work.

- **Family Medical Leave Act:** Generally, companies with fifty or more employees must provide eligible employees twelve weeks of unpaid time off with job protection to care for a family member. A few companies offer paid family leave for their caregiving employees.

- **Other benefits:** Your employer might provide senior care benefits such as seminars/webinars, temporary backup care, expert assistance, and eldercare referrals. Some employers also offer on-site care advisors and support groups.

- **Approach your manager:** It's best to talk directly with your manager and explain those late arrivals and urgent phone calls yourself. Try to work out a plan to handle your job and caregiving responsibilities at the same time.

- **Get human resources on board:** If you need to take a leave or adjust your schedule, speak with human resources to make that happen. If your employer doesn't offer eldercare benefits, be an advocate for yourself as well as for others in the same boat.

Caring for Someone with Dementia

Challenges for the Person with Dementia

- Has limited attention span and trouble following conversations
- Forgets names of objects or familiar people
- Experiences difficulty with multiple-step instructions
- Frequently repeats stories and familiar words
- Loses train of thought
- Exhibits sudden changes in mood
- Reverts back to a native language

Caregiver Strategies

- Understand problem behavior as an expression of an unmet need (hunger, pain, fatigue, frustration).

- Speak clearly and directly in a calm and caring manner.

- Refer to loved ones with dementia by name, and in their presence avoid speaking about them to others in the third person.

- Be patient and speak slowly in an adult tone of voice.

- Use direct eye contact and a warm, caring touch.

- Don't argue about reality or draw attention to inaccuracies.

- Find creative ways to engage through music, art, and movement.

- Utilize supports—the Alzheimer's Association has a twenty-four-hour helpline.

- Recognize that it's okay to use humor, which can be helpful and healing.

Doctor's Appointment Checklist

What should you bring?

- Written list of questions about new and ongoing concerns
- A notebook, laptop, or smart phone to record information during the visit
- Any mobility assistance an elder may need
- List of over-the-counter and prescription medications (including dosages) as well as vitamins and herbal supplements
- List of medical conditions, past and present
- Information about relevant family medical history
- List of other physicians and healthcare providers caring for your parent

- Information from other providers, if it has not been sent ahead of time
- Up-to-date insurance information and personal identification
- Legal documents such as a healthcare proxy, do-not-resuscitate order, HIPAA release form
- Other essentials such as glasses and hearing aids
- Beverages and snacks, in case you have a long wait

If you are unable to attend the appointment, consider hiring an aging life care professional who can advocate on behalf of your parent, ask the right questions, and update family members with important information following the visit.

What to Ask When Choosing a Nursing Home

- Is the nursing home Medicare/Medicaid-certified?
- What are the rates for private and semi-private rooms?
- What is and is not included in the daily rate?
- How is the plan of care created for each resident?
- Are families included in the care planning process?
- How frequently does staff check on residents?
- Are there specific resident conditions that the facility is not equipped to handle (for example, physical or verbal aggression)?
- Do residents have a choice in what time they wake up and go to sleep?
- Are there amenities such as cable TV, beauty parlor, library, and store?

- Is there a choice of menu and flexibility regarding times that residents eat?

- What types of recreational opportunities are offered, including activities and trips?

- Are background checks performed on all staff?

- Does direct care staff receive specialized training to care for dementia residents?

- Are there religious/spiritual programs in the facility?

- How long has the nursing home management team been in place?

- Is there a licensed doctor on staff, and how frequently are residents medically evaluated?

- Are residents allowed to see their primary care physicians and other medical providers?

- How long will a bed be held if the resident has Medicaid and is hospitalized?

- Have there been any recent deficiencies cited in state inspection surveys? If so, what were the deficiencies and how has the nursing home addressed them?

What to Ask When Choosing an Assisted Living Community

- Does the residence require an entrance fee?
- What does the monthly baseline fee include?
- What are the costs and availability of nonmedical home care?
- Are residents required to have renter's insurance?
- What additional services are offered for an extra fee, such as linens, laundry, and transportation?
- Is there a written care plan for each resident?
- Does the residence provide memory care and other specialized programs?
- Are there licensed staff who can administer medication?
- Does the residence have a nurse available 24/7?

- What meals are included and where are they served?

- Are there activities and events and is transportation included?

- What security measures are in place?

- Are calls for assistance responded to quickly?

- What is included in a sample contract and resident bill of rights?

- Under what circumstance would a resident have to leave the facility?

What to Ask When Choosing a Nonmedical Home Care Agency

- Does the agency meet state licensure requirements?

- How does the agency match caregivers with clients?

- What happens if a caregiver is not a good match? Can you request a change?

- Does the agency conduct background checks on all staff?

- Is staff bonded (insured against theft or loss in a home)?

- Do caregivers receive specialized training for Alzheimer's/dementia care and other disease-specific populations?

- Does the same caregiver attend to a client or is there a rotation?

- What if a caregiver does not show up? How quickly can the agency find a replacement?
- What is the hourly rate for a caregiver?
- Is there a contract you can review before choosing the agency?
- Is there a minimum number of hours required per day?
- Are there circumstances when overtime rates apply?
- Can caregivers drive clients to medical appointments and errands?
- Will caregivers use their own car or a client's vehicle?
- Does the agency ensure that caregivers have a safe driving record?
- How is communication handled between caregivers when there are multiple shifts?
- Does the agency have a nurse who develops and oversees a care plan?
- How often are care plans updated and do family members have input?
- How are after-hours phone calls handled?
- What procedures are in place in the event of an emergency?

Notes

ONE
The Journey Begins

1. Barbara Sadick, "A Remedy for the Looming Geriatrician Shortage," *Wall Street Journal*, June 8, 2014, accessed March 7, 2017, www.wsj.com/articles/a-remedy-for-the-looming-geriatrician-shortage-1402001802.

2. Marcy Cottrell Houle, "An Aging Population, without the Doctors to Match," *New York Times*, September 22, 2015, accessed March 7, 2017, http://www.nytimes.com/2015/09/23/opinion/an-aging-population-without-the-doctors-to-match.html?_r=0.

3. Elisabeth Kübler-Ross, *On Death and Dying* (New York: Simon & Schuster/Touchstone, 1969).

4. Alzheimer's Association, "2011 Alzheimer's Disease Facts and Figures," *Alzheimer's & Dementia* 7, no. 2 (2011): 208–44.

5. National Alliance for Caregiving and AARP, "Caregiving in the U.S.," June 2015, accessed March 7, 2017, http://www.caregiving.org/wp-content/uploads/2015/05/2015_CaregivingintheUS_Executive-Summary-June-4_WEB.pdf.

6. Susannah Fox and Joanna Brenner, "Family Caregivers Online," Pew Research Center, July 12, 2012, accessed March 7, 2017, http://www.pewinternet.org/2012/07/12/family-caregivers-online/.

THREE

The Parent Who Rejects Help

1. Insurance Institute for Highway Safety, "Older Drivers: Older People, 2013," accessed March 7, 2017, http://www.iihs.org/iihs/topics /t/older-drivers/fatalityfacts/older-people/2013.

2. Jacopo Prisco, "Why UPS Trucks (Almost) Never Turn Left," *CNN*, February 23, 2017, accessed March 7, 2017, http://www.cnn.com/ 2017/02/16/world/ups-trucks-no-left-turns/.

3. SeniorDriving.AAA.com, "Professional Assessment," accessed March 7, 2017, http://seniordriving.aaa.com/evaluate-your-driving-ability/ professional-assessment/.

4. AARP, "AARP Driver Safety," accessed March 7, 2017, http://www .aarp.org/ws/EO/driver-safety-programs/.

5. Erik Erikson, *Childhood and Society* (New York: Norton, 1950).

6. Erik H. Erikson, *The Life Cycle Completed: Extended Version with New Chapters on the Ninth Stage of Development by Joan M. Erikson* (New York: Norton, 1998); U.S. Census Bureau, "2010 Census Shows 65 and Older Population Growing Faster Than Total U.S. Population," November 30, 2011, accessed March 7, 2017, https://www.census .gov/newsroom/releases/archives/2010_census/cb11-cn192.html.

7. P. S. Ciechanowski, W. J. Katon, J. E. Russo, and E. A. Walker, "The Patient-Provider Relationship: Attachment Theory and Adherence to Treatment in Diabetes," *American Journal of Psychiatry* 158, no. 1 (2001): 29–35.

8. Centers for Disease Control, "The State of Aging & Health in America, 2013," accessed March 7, 2017, http://www.cdc.gov/aging/ pdf/state-aging-health-in-america-2013.pdf.

FOUR

Good, Bad, and Nonexistent Siblings

1. AARP and the National Alliance for Caregiving, "Caregiving in the U.S."

2. Ibid.

3. Elizabeth Bernstein, "Sibling Rivalry Grows Up: Adult Brothers and Sisters Are Masters at Digs; Finding a Way to a Truce," *Wall Street Journal*, March 20, 2012, accessed March 8, 2017, http://www.wsj.com /articles/SB10001424052702304724404577291432292777576.

4. Karl Pillemer and J. Jill Sutior, "Who Provides Care? A Prospective

Study of Caregiving among Adult Siblings," *Gerontologist* 54, no. 4 (2014): 589–98.

5. L. M. Amaro and K. I. Miller, "Discussion of Care, Contribution, and Perceived (In) Gratitude in the Family Caregiver and Sibling Relationship," *Personal Relationships* 23, no. 1 (2016): 98–110.

6. Ibid.

7. Karl Pillemer, J. Jill Suitor, Catherine Riffin, and Meagan Gilligan, "Adult Children's Problems and Mothers' Well-being: Does Parental Favoritism Matter?" *Research on Aging*, October 2015, accessed March 8, 2017, http://journals.sagepub.com/doi/10.1177/0164027515611464.

8. Gretchen Livingston, "Family Size among Mothers," Pew Research Center, May 7, 2015, accessed March 8, 2017, http://www.pewsocialtrends.org/2015/05/07/family-size-among-mothers/.

9. Deb Song, "Cracking under the Cultural Code," Rush University Medical Center, December 18, 2015, accessed March 8, 2017, https://www.rush.edu/news/cracking-under-cultural-code.

10. Francine Russo, *They're Your Parents, Too! How Siblings Can Survive Their Parents' Aging without Driving Each Other Crazy* (New York: Bantam, 2010), 108.

11. Victor Cicirelli, *Sibling Relations across the Life Span* (New York: Springer US, 1995).

FIVE

What Does Care Cost, and Who Pays?

1. James. B. Stewart, "When Family Fortunes Beget Vicious Power Struggles," *New York Times*, February 11, 2016, accessed March 8, 2017, https://www.nytimes.com/2016/02/12/business/media/when-family-fortunes-beget-vicious-power-struggles.html?_r=0.

2. Russell Heimlich, "Baby Boomers Retire," Pew Research Center, December 29, 2010, accessed March 8, 2017, http://www.pewresearch.org/fact-tank/2010/12/29/baby-boomers-retire/.

3. LongTermCare.gov, "Who Needs Care?" last modified February 21, 2017, accessed March 8, 2017, https://longtermcare.acl.gov/the-basics/who-needs-care.html.

4. Susan Reinhard, Lynn Friss Feinberg, Rita Choula, and Ari Houser, "Valuing the Invaluable: 2015 Update," AARP Public Policy Institute, July 2015, accessed March 7, 2017, http://www.aarp.org/content/dam/aarp/ppi/2015/valuing-the-invaluable-2015-update-new.pdf.

5. Genworth, "2016 Genworth Annual Cost of Care Study," last up-dated June 22, 2016, accessed March 8, 2017, https://www.genworth.com/about-us/industry-expertise/cost-of-care.html.

6. Jeff Charles Goldsmith, *The Long Baby Boom: An Optimistic Vision for a Graying Generation* (Baltimore: Johns Hopkins University Press, 2008).

7. National Public Radio, Robert Wood Johnson Foundation, and Harvard School of Public Health, "Retirement and Health," September 1, 2011, accessed March 8, 2017, http://www.rwjf.org/en/library/research/2011/09/retirement-and-health-poll.html.

8. David Solie, *How to Say It to Seniors: Closing the Communication Gap with Our Elders* (New York: Prentice Hall, 2004).

9. MACPAC, "MACStates: Medicaid and CHIP Program Statistics," June 2014, accessed March 15, 2017, https://www.macpac.gov/wp-content/uploads/2015/01/2014_06_MACStats.pdf; Medicaid.gov, "December 2016 Medicaid and CHIP Enrollment Data Highlights," December 2016, accessed March 15, 2017, https://www.medicaid.gov/medicaid/program-information/medicaid-and-chip-enrollment-data/report-highlights/index.html.

10. CMS, "Medicare Enrollment–National Trends 1966–2013," 2014, accessed March 15, 2017, https://www.cms.gov/Research-Statistics-Data-and-Systems/Statistics-Trends-and-Reports/MedicareEnrpts/Downloads/SMI2013.pdf; CMS, "Medicare Enrollment Dashboard," December 2016, accessed March 15, 2017, https://www.cms.gov/Research-Statistics-Data-and-Systems/Statistics-Trends-and-Reports/Dashboard/Medicare-Enrollment/Enrollment%20Dashboard.html.

11. CMS, "History: CMS' Program History," last modified January 1, 2017, accessed March 15, 2017, https://www.cms.gov/About-CMS/Agency-Information/History/index.html?redirect=/history/.

12. Chuck Rainville, Laura Skufca, and Laura Mehegan, "Family Caregiving and Out-of-Pocket Costs: 2016 Report," AARP, November 2016, accessed March 10, 2017, http://www.aarp.org/content/dam/aarp/research/surveys_statistics/ltc/2016/family-caregiving-cost-survey-res-ltc.pdf.

13. Genworth, "Cost of Care."

14. Ibid.

15. Ibid.

SIX

The Care Maze

1. Stephen Jencks, Mark Williams, and Eric Coleman, " Rehospitalizations among Patients in the Medicare Fee-for-Service Program," *New England Journal of Medicine* 360 (2009): 1418–28.
2. Robert Kane, *The Good Caregiver: A One-of-a-Kind Compassionate Resource for Anyone Caring for an Aging Loved One* (New York: Penguin Group, 2011).
3. Susan Reinhard, Carol Levine, and Sarah Samis, *Home Alone: Family Caregivers Providing Complex Chronic Care*, AARP and United Hospital Fund, October 2012, accessed March 10, 2017, http://www.aarp .org/content/dam/aarp/research/public_policy_institute/health/ home-alone-family-caregivers-providing-complex-chronic-care-rev -AARP-ppi-health.pdf.
4. Ibid.
5. Elaine Ryan, "The CARE Act: Helping Family Caregivers from Hospital to Home," AARP, March 7, 2016, accessed June 21, 2016, http://blog.aarp.org/2016/03/07/the-care-act-helping-family-care givers-from-hospital-to-home/.
6. Medicare Interactive, "Original Medicare Appeals if Your Care Is Ending (Hospital, SNF, CORF, Hospice, Home Health Care)," accessed March 10, 2017, http://www.medicareinteractive.org/get-an swers/medicare-rights-and-appeals/original-medicare-appeals/ original-medicare-appeals-if-your-care-is-ending-hospital-snf -corf-hospice-home-health-care.
7. AARP Public Policy Institute, "Chronic Care: A Call to Action for Health Care Reform," 2009, accessed March 10, 2017, http://assets .aarp.org/rgcenter/health/beyond_50_hcr.pdf.

SEVEN

Making Work Work

1. AARP and ReAct, "Determining the Return on Investment: Supportive Policies for Employee Caregivers," April 2016, accessed March 14, 2017, http://respectcaregivers.org/wp-content/uploads/ 2016/04/AARP-ROI-Report-FINAL-4.1.16.pdf.
2. Lynn Feinberg and Rita Choula, "Understanding the Impact of Family Caregiving on Work," AARP Public Policy Institute, October 2012, accessed March 14, 2017, http://www.aarp.org/content/

dam/aarp/research/public_policy_institute/ltc/2012/understand
ing-impact-family-caregivingwork-AARP-ppi-ltc.pdf.

3. MetLife Mature Market Institute, "The MetLife Study of Caregiving
Costs to Working Caregivers: Double Jeopardy for Baby Boomers
Caring for Their Parents," 2011, accessed March 14, 2017, https://
www.metlife.com/assets/cao/mmi/publications/studies/2011/High
lights/mmi-caregiving-costs-working-caregivers-highlights.pdf.

4. Elizabeth Mendes, "Most Caregivers Look After Elderly Parent, Invest
a Lot of Time," Gallup Healthways Wellbeing Survey, July 28, 2011,
accessed March 14, 2017, http://www.gallup.com/poll/148682/care
givers-look-elderly-parent-invest-lot-time.aspx.

5. Cynthia Calvert, "Caregivers in the Workplace: Family Responsibilities Discrimination Litigation Update, 2016," UC Hasting College
of Law, Work Life Law, 2016, accessed March 14, 2017, http://www
.worklifelaw.org/pubs/FRDupdate2016.pdf.

6. Ibid.

7. Ibid.

8. AARP and ReAct, "Determining the Return on Investment."

9. United States Department of Labor Wage and Hour Division, Family and Medical Leave Act, accessed March 14, 2017, https://www
.dol.gov/whd/fmla/.

10. Brigid Schulte, "Aging Population Prompts More Employers to
Offer Elder-Care Benefits to Workers," *Washington Post*, November
16, 2014, accessed July 18, 2016, https://www.washingtonpost.com/
local/aging-population-prompts-more-employers-to-offer-elder
-care-benefits-to-workers/2014/11/16/25f9c8e6–6847–11e4-a31c
-77759fc1eacc_story.html.

11. National Alliance for Caregiving, University of Pittsburgh Institute
on Aging, and MetLife Mature Market Institute, "The MetLife
Study of Working Caregivers and Employer Health Costs: New
Insights and Innovations for Reducing Health Care Costs for Employers," February 2010, accessed March 14, 2017, https://www
.metlife.com/assets/cao/mmi/publications/studies/2010/mmi
-working-caregivers-employers-health-care-costs.pdf.

12. National Alliance for Caregiving and AARP, "Caregiving in the
U.S."

EIGHT

The Art of Connection

1. Alzheimer's Association, "2017 Alzheimer's Disease Facts and Figures," accessed June 5, 2017, http://www.alz.org/facts/.
2. Ibid.
3. Ibid.
4. Dr. Bill Thomas, *Life's Most Dangerous Game, P.L.A.Y. Book* (AARP, 2016) (booklet distributed at Disrupt Dementia tour).
5. John Zeisel, *I'm Still Here: A Breakthrough Approach to Understanding Someone Living with Alzheimer's* (New York: Penguin Group, 2009).
6. Oliver Sacks, *Musicophilia: Tale of Music and the Brain* (New York: Knopf, 2007).
7. Joanne Koenig Coste, *Learning to Speak Alzheimer's: A Groundbreaking Approach for Everyone Dealing with the Disease* (Boston: Houghton Mifflin, 2003).
8. Alzheimer's Association, letter to Commission on Long-Term Care, August 16, 2013, accessed March 14, 2017, http://www.alz.org/national/documents/Long-Term-Care-Commission-8-16-13.pdf.
9. Nancy Mace and Peter Rabins, *The 36-Hour Day: A Family Guide to Caring for People Who Have Alzheimer Disease, Other Dementias, and Memory Loss*, 6th ed. (Baltimore: Johns Hopkins University Press, 2017).
10. Alzheimer's Association, "Younger/Early Onset Alzheimer's & Dementia," accessed March 14, 2017, http://www.alz.org/alzheimers_disease_early_onset.asp.

NINE

Caring for the Parent Who Couldn't Care for You

1. Jooyoung Kong and Sara Moorman, "Caring for My Abuser: Childhood Maltreatment and Caregiver Depression," *Gerontologist* 55, no. 4 (2015): 656–66.
2. Harry Haroutunian, *Not as Prescribed: Recognizing and Facing Alcohol and Drug Misuse in Older Adults; A Guide for Families and Caregivers* (Center City, MN: Hazeldon, 2016).
3. Ibid.
4. Eleanor Cade, *Taking Care of Parents Who Didn't Take Care of You: Making Peace with Aging Parents* (Center City, MN: Hazeldon, 2002).

5. Mark Agronin, "Struggling with an Abusive Aging Parent," *New York Times, New Old Age*, August 13, 2012, accessed March 14, 2017, http://newoldage.blogs.nytimes.com/2012/08/13/struggling-with-an-abusive-aging-parent/?_r=0.

6. Patrick J. Kennedy and Stephen Fried, *A Common Struggle: A Personal Journey through the Past and Future of Mental Illness and Addiction* (New York: Blue Rider, 2015), 185.

7. Richard Friedman, "When Parents Are Too Toxic to Tolerate," *New York Times*, October 19, 2009, accessed March 14, 2017, http://www.nytimes.com/2009/10/20/health/20mind.html?_r=1.

8. Craig Reaves, "Ask the Expert: Parental Support and the Law," *New York Times, New Old Age*, February 26, 2010, accessed March 14, 2017, http://newoldage.blogs.nytimes.com/2010/02/26/ask-the-expert-parental-support-and-the-law/.

9. National Alliance for Caregiving, Mental Health America, and National Alliance for Mental Illness, "On Pins and Needles: Caregivers of Adults with Mental Illness," February 2016, accessed March 14, 2017, http://www.caregiving.org/wp-content/uploads/2016/02/NAC_Mental_Illness_Study_2016_FINAL_WEB.pdf.

TEN

How to Care for Ourselves Too

1. American Psychological Association. "Stress in America: Our Health at Risk," 2012, accessed March 14, 2017, http://www.apa.org/news/press/releases/stress/2011/final-2011.pdf.

2. Merriam-Webster dictionary definition of *burnout*, accessed March 14, 2017, www.merriam-webster.com/dictionary/burnout.

3. Barry J. Jacobs, *The Emotional Survival Guide for Caregivers: Looking After Yourself and Your Family While Helping an Aging Parent* (New York: Guilford, 2006).

4. Hugh Marriott, *The Selfish Pig's Guide to Caring: How to Cope with the Emotional and Practical Aspects of Caring for Someone* (Boston: Little, Brown Book Group, 2012).

5. Ron Acierno et al., "Prevalence and Correlates of Emotional, Physical, Sexual, and Financial Abuse and Potential Neglect in the United States: The National Elder Mistreatment Study," *American Journal of Public Health* 100, no. 2 (2010): 292–97.

6. Scott Beach et al., "Risk Factors for Potentially Harmful Informal

Caregiver Behavior," *Journal of the American Geriatrics Society* 53, no. 2 (2005): 255–61.

7. National Alliance for Caregiving and AARP, "Caregiving in the U.S."

8. R. Schulz and S. Beach, "Caregiving as a Risk Factor for Mortality: The Caregiver Health Effects Study," *JAMA* 282, no. 23 (1999): 2215–19.

ELEVEN

Letting Go

1. Barry Jacobs, "Feeling Relief (and Guilt) at Caregiving's End," AARP, accessed March 14, 2017, http://www.aarp.org/home-family/caregiving/info-2015/relief-and-guilt-when-caregiving-ends.html.

2. Atul Gawande, *Being Mortal: Medicine and What Matters in the End* (New York: Metropolitan Books, 2014).

3. Stephanie Armour, "End-of-Life Discussions Will Be Reimbursed by Medicare," *Wall Street Journal*, October 30, 2015, accessed March 14, 2017, http://www.wsj.com/articles/end-of-life-discussions-will-be-reimbursed-by-medicare-1446240608.

4. National Hospice and Palliative Care Organization, "NHPCO's Facts and Figures: Hospice Care in America," 2015, accessed March 14, 2017, http://www.nhpco.org/sites/default/files/public/Statistics_Research/2015_Facts_Figures.pdf.

5. L. L. Cohen, "Racial/Ethnic Disparities in Hospice Care: A Systematic Review," *Journal of Palliative Medicine* 11, no. 5 (2008): 763–68.

6. National Hospice and Palliative Care Organization, "Facts and Figures."

7. *This American Death*, documentary film written and directed by Susan Austin, produced by Lorielle Mallue, 2015.

8. Roz Chast, *Can't We Talk about Something More Pleasant? A Memoir* (New York: Bloomsbury USA, 2014).

TWELVE

Moving Forward, Looking Back

1. AARP and HITLAB, "Caregivers and Technology: What They Want and Need; A Guide for Innovators—Research from a Nation-

ally Representative Sample of America's 40 Million Family Caregivers," April 2016, accessed March 14, 2017, http://www.aarp.org/con tent/dam/aarp/home-and-family/personal-technology/2016/04/ Caregivers-and-Technology-AARP.pdf.

2. Donald Redfoot, Lynn Feinberg, and Ari Houser, "The Aging of the Baby Boom and the Growing Care Gap: A Look at Future Declines in the Availability of Family Caregivers," AARP Policy Institute, August 2013, accessed March 14, 2017, http://www.aarp.org/content/ dam/aarp/research/public_policy_institute/ltc/2013/baby-boom -and-the-growing-care-gap-insight-AARP-ppi-ltc.pdf.

3. V. A. Freedman and B. C. Spillman, "Disability and Care Needs among Older Americans," *Milbank Quarterly* 92, no. 3 (2014): 509–41.

4. Steven Dawson, "The Direct Care Workforce—Raising the Floor of Job Quality," *Generations* (Spring 2016), 38, 39.

5. Andy Newman, "Therapy Cats for Dementia Patients, Batteries Included," *New York Times*, December 15, 2016, accessed March 14, 2017, http://www.nytimes.com/2016/12/15/nyregion/robotic-therapy -cats-dementia.html?_r=0.

6. National Opinion Research Center and the Associated Press, "Long Term Care in America: Expectations and Reality," March 2014, accessed March 14, 2017, http://www.longtermcarepoll.org/PDFs/ LTC%202014/AP-NORC-Long-Term%20Care%20in%20Amer ica_FINAL%20WEB.pdf.

Resources

Aging

- AARP (www.aarp.org)
- Administration on Aging (www.aoa.gov)
- Aging in Place Technology Watch (www.ageinplacetech.com)
- Aging with Dignity (www.agingwithdignity.org)
- American Association for Geriatric Psychiatry (www.aagponline.org)
- American Geriatrics Society (www.americangeriatrics.org)
- American Geriatrics Society Foundation Health in Aging (www.healthinaging.org)
- American Society on Aging (www.asaging.org)
- SAGE: Services and Advocacy for Gay, Lesbian, Bisexual & Transgender Elders (www.sageusa.org)

Caregiving and Care Providers

- Adult Children of Aging Parents Community (www.acapcommunity.org)

- Aging Life Care Association (www.aginglifecare.org)
- ARCH National Respite Network (www.archrespite.org)
- Area Agency on Aging (www.n4a.org)
- Argentum (www.argentum.org)
- Care.com (www.care.com)
- Caregiver Action Network (www.caregiveraction.org)
- *Caregiver Magazine* (www.caregiver.com)
- CaringBridge (www.caringbridge.org)
- Elder Care Locator (www.eldercare.gov)
- Family Caregiver Alliance: National Center on Caregiving (www.caregiver.org/national-center-caregiving)
- Leading Age (www.leadingage.org)
- Lotsa Helping Hands (www.lotsahelpinghands.com)
- National Adult Day Services Association (www.nadsa.org)
- National Adult Protective Services Association (www.napsa -now.org)
- National Alliance for Caregiving (www.caregiving.org)
- National Association of Social Workers (www.socialworkers .org)
- National Center for Assisted Living (www.ncal.org)
- National Council on Aging (www.ncoa.org)
- Program of All-Inclusive Care for the Elderly (www.npaonline .org/pace-you)
- ReACT (Respecting a Caregiver's Time) (www.respectcare givers.org)
- Self-Compassion (www.selfcompassion.org)
- Village to Village Network (www.vtvnetwork.org)

Disease-Specific Information

- ALS Association (www.als.org)
- Alzheimer's Association (www.alz.org)
- American Cancer Society (www.cancer.org)
- American Diabetes Association (www.diabetes.org)

- American Heart Association (www.heart.org)
- American Stroke Association (www.strokeassociation.org)
- Centers for Disease Control (www.cdc.gov)
- National Alliance on Mental Illness (www.nami.org)
- National Parkinson's Foundation (www.parkinson.org)
- UsAgainstAlzheimer's (www.usagainstalzheimers.org)

Driving

- AAA (www.seniordriving.aaa.com)
- AAA Foundation for Traffic Safety (www.aaafoundation.org)
- AARP Driving Safety Program (www.aarp.org/families/driver _safety)
- Clearinghouse for Older Road User Safety: ChORUS (www .roadsafeseniors.org)

End of Life Care

- The Conversation Project (www.theconversationproject.org)
- Death Café (www.deathcafe.com)
- National Association of Home Care and Hospice (www.nahc .org)
- National Hospice and Palliative Care Organization (www.nhp co.org)

Financial and Legal

- American Association for Long-Term Care Insurance (www .aaltci.org)
- Benefits Checkup (www.benefitscheckup.org)
- Center for Medicare Advocacy (www.medicareadvocacy.org)
- Elder Law Answers (www.elderlawanswers.com)
- Genworth Annual Cost of Care Study (www.genworth.com/ about-us/industry-expertise/cost-of-care.html)

- LawHelp.org (www.lawhelp.org)
- Long Term Care Information from U.S. Department of Health and Human Services (www.longtermcare.gov)
- Mediate.com (www.mediate.com)
- Medicaid (www.Medicaid.gov)
- Medicare (www.Medicare.gov)
- Medicare Rights Center (www.MedicareInteractive.org)
- National Academy of Elder Law Attorneys (www.naela.org)
- National Long Term Care Ombudsman Resources Center (www.ltcombudsman.org)
- Social Security Administration (www.ssa.gov)
- True Link Financial (www.truelinkfinancial.com)
- Veterans Benefits Administration, U.S. Department of Veterans Affairs (www.va.gov)
- Veterans Financial (www.veteransfinancial.com)

Recommended Further Reading

Cade, Eleanor. *Taking Care of Parents Who Didn't Take Care of You: Making Peace with Aging Parents.* Center City, MN: Hazelden, 2002.

Chast, Roz. *Can't We Talk about Something More Pleasant? A Memoir.* New York: Bloomsbury USA, 2014.

Comer, Meryl. *Slow Dancing with a Stranger: Lost and Found in the Age of Alzheimer's.* New York: HarperCollins, 2014.

Coste, Joanne Koenig. *Learning to Speak Alzheimer's: A Groundbreaking Approach for Everyone Dealing with the Disease.* Boston: Houghton Mifflin, 2003.

Gawande, Atul. *Being Mortal: Medicine and What Matters in the End.* New York: Metropolitan Books, 2014.

Gross, Jane. *A Bittersweet Season: Caring for Our Aging Parents and Ourselves.* New York: Knopf, 2011.

Haroutunian, Harry. *Not as Prescribed: Recognizing and Facing Alcohol and Drug Misuse in Older Adults; A Guide for Families and Caregivers.* Center City, MN: Hazelden, 2016.

Jacobs, Barry J. *The Emotional Survival Guide for Caregivers: Looking After Yourself and Your Family While Helping an Aging Parent.* New York: Guilford, 2006.

Kane, Robert. *The Good Caregiver: A One-of-a-Kind Compassionate Resource for Anyone Caring for an Aging Loved One*. New York: Penguin Group, 2011.

Kane, Robert, and Joan West. *It Shouldn't Have to Be This Way: The Failure of Long-Term Care*. Nashville: Vanderbilt University Press, 2005.

Kennedy, Patrick J., and Stephen Fried. *A Common Struggle: A Personal Journey through the Past and Future of Mental Illness and Addiction*. New York: Blue Rider, 2016.

Loverde, Joy. *The Complete Eldercare Planner: Where to Start, Which Questions to Ask, and How to Find Help*. New York: Three Rivers, 2009.

Mace, Nancy, and Peter Rabins. *The 36-Hour Day: A Family Guide to Caring for People Who Have Alzheimer Disease, Other Dementias, and Memory Loss*. 6th ed. Baltimore: Johns Hopkins University Press, 2017.

Marriott, Hugh. *The Selfish Pig's Guide to Caring: How to Cope with the Emotional and Practical Aspects of Caring for Someone*. Boston: Little, Brown Book Group, 2012.

Pfeiffer, Eric. *Caregiving in Alzheimer's and Other Dementias*. New Haven: Yale University Press, 2015.

Russo, Francine. *They're Your Parents, Too! How Siblings Can Survive Their Parents' Aging without Driving Each Other Crazy*. New York: Bantam, 2010.

Solie, David. *How to Say It to Seniors: Closing the Communication Gap with Our Elders*. New York: Prentice Hall, 2004.

Span, Paula. *When the Time Comes: Families with Aging Parents Share Their Struggles and Solutions*. New York: Springboard, 2009.

Zeisel, John. *I'm Still Here: A Breakthrough Approach to Understanding Someone Living with Alzheimer's*. New York: Penguin Group, 2009.

Acknowledgments

The initial idea of writing this book was not my own. One day, when I was discussing my annual performance goals at Care.com, Donna Levin, my boss and the company's co-founder, enthusiastically suggested I write a book. Given everything on my plate at the time, this seemed like an impossible feat, and I let it go. But gradually the idea took hold, and many years later a book was born. I owe an enormous debt of gratitude to Sheila Marcelo, CEO and founder of Care.com, and the people at the company who encouraged and supported me along the way, including Josh Fine, Nancy Bushkin, Diane Musi, Erica Scheik, Latoya Murphy, Elizabeth Tutschek Scott, Jill McNamara, and the entire senior care team.

Writing a book truly takes a village, and I was blessed to have one. It was my good fortune to find Linda Konner, a wise and talented literary agent, whose efforts led to a book deal with a distinguished publisher. I am extremely grateful to Jean Thomson Black, senior executive editor of Yale University Press, Margaret Otzel, Robin DuBlanc, Michael Dineen, and to the entire team at Yale for their support and dedication to this project, and to Elizabeth Shreve, my savvy and seasoned publicist.

I was greatly honored that former U.S. representative Patrick J. Kennedy agreed to write the foreword. Through dedication to public service and a commitment to compassionate policy, Patrick and his father, the late senator Ted Kennedy, have made significant and lasting contributions to the American family.

Emily Saltz and Harry Margolis generously lent their professional expertise through numerous interviews and edits. Allison Cook served as my invaluable and trusted research assistant. Belinda Hulin provided incisive feedback on early drafts of the manuscript.

This book would not have been possible without the many family caregivers who generously shared their personal experiences with me. Their stories and deep understanding of the burdens and benefits of caregiving brought this book to life.

My greatest appreciation goes to my family. My brother Keith Oppenheim, former correspondent for CNN and now professor at Champlain College, was one of my most trusted reviewers. His recollections of our shared family history, along with his irreverent humor and keen insights, were extremely helpful and kept up my spirits. My sister Lisa Berzins, a prominent clinical psychologist, taught me about the importance of self-compassion and how it can uplift and enlighten caregivers. Much of the inspiration for this book comes from my mother Adele Oppenheim, an extraordinary caregiver, and my father Henry Oppenheim, who boldly embraced life throughout his years of dementia.

My adult children were my constant cheering squad and often the fuel that kept me going. Eric read many early drafts and gave me feedback with smiley-faced encouragement. Daniel served as the grammar police and teased me about my inexplicable use of commas and numerous challenges with end-notes. Rebecca taught me to embrace the creative process and accept that it sometimes feels like a "hot mess." The biggest thank-you goes to my husband David, who helped me discover my voice as a writer. He believed from the get-go that I could write a book and accomplish what initially felt like mission impossible. I am grateful to have had such incredible support to guide me through this humbling and exhilarating journey.

Index

AAA (American Automobile Association), 45

AAAs. *See* Area Agencies on Aging

AARP (American Association of Retired Persons): on advocacy, 141; CARE Act proposed by, 131; driver safety program from, 45; *Home Alone* study conducted by, 130

abuse: by caregivers, 54, 218–21; elder abuse, 218–21; sexual, 188; substance abuse, 187–90, 193–94, 197

acceptance: of caregiver limitations, xix, 25–26, 31–32, 57–58, 266; of dementia diagnosis, 4, 10–12; of help, 20, 37, 40–41, 51, 55–56; radical strategy for, 25; of sibling limitations, 70, 84

adaptability of caregivers, 35

addiction, 188–90, 194–95, 197, 226

Administration on Aging (AoA), 134–35

adult day care, 110–11

Adult Protective Services, 220

advance care planning, 236, 244–45

advocacy, 141–42, 163

African Americans, caregiving views among, 52

aging in place, 22, 114–15, 253–54

Aging in Place Technology Watch, 253

Aging Life Care Association, 19, 67

aging life care professionals, 19–20, 57, 83, 115, 134, 276

About the Author

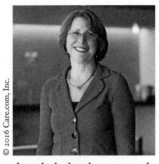

© 2016 Care.com, Inc.

Jody Gastfriend, LICSW, is the vice president of senior care for Care.com, the world's largest online destination for finding and managing family care. As a licensed clinical social worker with more than twenty-five years of experience, Jody knows the challenges and struggles of family caregivers, having for more than a decade helped manage the care of her own father, who had dementia. Jody has held a wide range of leadership positions, including director of social service in a community hospital, chief operating officer of a home care agency, and consultant to hospitals and long-term care facilities. Jody has lectured widely to family caregivers, HR administrators, healthcare professionals, and policy makers on topics ranging from eldercare and aging to work and family integration. A featured senior care expert for NBC, Fox News, AARP, and the *Wall Street Journal*, Jody is a contributor to the Huffington Post's Huff/Post50 section and has published numerous articles on caregiving and aging. Jody received her bachelor of arts, magna cum laude, from Tufts University, and her master's degree in social work from Simmons College School of Social Work.